Praise for *Metabolism Makeover*

"Finally . . . a much-needed antidote to the diet industry's 'eat less, exercise more' mantra! I love Megan's holistic body-and-mind approach to weight loss, and it's the approach that helped me finally break free of dieting and heal my metabolism. She also provides valuable tools for tapping into your subconscious for true behavior change and long-term results. A must read!"

—Katie Wells, founder of WellnessMama.com

"Megan is a breath of fresh air in the health-and-wellness space. She is so in tune with the body, and in an approachable way, she helps people learn what works best for them. It's not a one-size-fits-all when it comes to health and weight loss, and no one understands that better than Megan. I highly recommend adding *Metabolism Makeover* to your wellness tool kit."

—Lauryn Bosstick, founder of the Skinny Confidential brand and website

"Megan really nailed it by highlighting the importance of building healthy muscle, which is often overlooked in the weight-loss conversation. Great guidebook!"

—Dr. Gabrielle Lyon, founder of the Institute for Muscle-Centric Medicine

"Megan's comprehensive and relatable approach to improving metabolism is an absolute game changer for everyone frustrated with feeling stuck in the outdated nutrition philosophy of 'eat less, move more.'

Metabolism Makeover gives you the playbook necessary for finally feeling empowered and capable of achieving long-term results without feeling deprived!"

—Brigid Titgemeier, MS, RDN, LD, IFNCP, and founder of BeingBrigid Functional Nutrition

"If you care deeply about your overall health and well-being and want a guide that truly empowers you to finally conquer your weight management and mindset, put this book on your required-reading list. Megan breaks down the truth about a healthy metabolism and provides actionable steps to make true and lasting changes once and for all. This is a must read!"

—Tina Anderson, CEO and cofounder of Just Thrive

"I devoured this book. It made me laugh; it made me cry; it made me think and rethink. I will give this book to all the women in my life who need the sort of empowerment that comes from an educated, funny, and authentic professional. Megan's words are powerful and transformative, and they give readers the courage to embrace themselves as masterpieces AND works in progress. She teaches readers to sink deeply into the unapologetic realness of who they are in all their seasons of life."

—Dr. Erin Nitschke, ACE Health Coach, fitness nutrition specialist, and therapeutic exercise specialist

METABOLISM MAKEOVER

MEGAN HANSEN, RDN

METABOLISM MAKEOVER

Ditch the Diet, Train Your Brain, Drop the Weight **for Good**

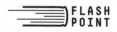

Published by Flashpoint Books™, Seattle
www.flashpointbooks.com

FLASH POINT

Edited and designed by Girl Friday Productions
www.girlfridayproductions.com

Cover design: Megan Katsanevakis
Project management: Mari Kesselring and Laura Dailey
Image credits: cover © istock/Saddako (cake); istock/t_kimura (spaghetti); istock/MiguelMalo (shrimp); istock/LauriPatterson (steak); istock/Андрей Ёлкин (forks); istock/urfinguss (avocado); shutterstock/Washdog (background)

ISBN (paperback): 978-1-736357-98-9
ISBN (ebook): 978-1-736324-35-6

Library of Congress Control Number: 2023901899

First edition

CONTENTS

HOW WE GOT HERE

I remember the (first) time I ate an entire jar of peanut butter on my bedroom floor.

I was 19 and in college, studying to become a dietitian. That semester, I was working on a class project that replicated how we'd walk a patient through a weight-loss program:

- Step 1: Determine how many calories the patient requires to maintain their current weight.
- Step 2: Determine the patient's goal weight based on their height, using a Hamwi ideal body weight chart.
- Step 3: Determine how large of a calorie deficit they'd have to sustain, based on how much weight they had to lose. Since 3,500 calories convert to one pound of body fat, one must sustain a 3,500-calorie deficit to lose one pound.
- Step 4: Create a calorie-intake goal (food!) and a calorie-output goal (cardio!). If the goal is to lose two pounds per week, the total deficit for the week would need to be 7,000 calories, or a 1,000-calorie deficit per day. This often would look like eating 500 fewer calories and doing enough cardio to burn 500 calories each day.
- Step 5: Track calorie intake and output in a food and exercise journal to stay on track.

- Step 6: Watch the weight come off precisely as it should, according to the above formulas.

Our assignment was to put ourselves through these calculations and keep a food journal for a period of time. In theory, this was a great idea because by experiencing what our patients would experience, we would easily be able to show them empathy and grace throughout this major life change.

We were given the option either to reduce our own calorie intake if we felt that we wanted to lose weight or to eat at a maintenance level of calorie intake (i.e., the number of calories your body needs to maintain its current weight). I chose the weight-loss route, because according to the ideal body weight charts we were using, I could lose another five pounds.

One night, after weeks of barely eating 1,200 calories and squeezing in 60-minute runs every day, I came home after eating dinner and was out-of-control starving. Ravenous.

I grabbed a jar of Jif peanut butter out of a roommate's cupboard and stuck my entire hand in it. And I didn't stop. I took down that peanut butter jar with my bare hands.

Afterward, I sat on the floor in a daze, wondering WTF just happened. I felt sick, gross, and embarrassed. My roommate was going to be pissed. Mostly, though, I felt the fear creep in as I started to add up the calories I'd just consumed. I got into bed and lay there, wondering how tomorrow I'd make up for all those extra calories I just ate. I could get up earlier to work out before class, skip breakfast, miss dinner and a night out with my roommates, or cut out carbs for the rest of the week.

None of these options would solve the actual problem, because the problem was never the calories—the problem was right inside my head. Overexercising and starving myself only made things worse by creating a constant obsession with food and my body. It also made me more hungry, which added fuel to the binge-restrict cycle I had found myself in. I could have saved myself years of playing out this scene over and over again if I had just asked myself why I'd do something as bizarre as manhandle a jar of peanut butter in the first place.

Instead, I spent the next five years doing strange things because of food. I skipped social events when I wouldn't have control over my food choices. I ate a roommate's Pop-Tarts in the closet late at night. I cut carbs out of my diet Monday through Thursday so that I could binge on vodka and gyros all weekend long. I took a can of beets to a kegger to curb my hunger so I wouldn't eat the pizza. To sum up, I lived in a constant cycle of shame about who I was—a person who was studying to help people with food and their weight but who had no control over food or her own weight.

I finished college with a 3.9 GPA and was placed in my first-choice dietetic internship program, where I graduated at the top of my class and passed my boards on the first try. I was a brand-new, model dietitian who had completed her studies with a 25-pound weight gain and a severely disordered relationship with food and her body.

I'm not quite sure what got into me as I approached rock bottom with my eating and weight issues, but shortly after passing my boards and becoming a registered dietitian nutritionist, I came across an article that claimed lifting weights for just a few hours per week was a more effective weight-loss strategy than hitting the treadmill every day. This made no sense to me, because an hour of cardio easily burned more calories than an hour of weight lifting. After reading the entire article, I thought the whole thing sounded suspicious, but *man*, I hated running.

What happened next changed the entire trajectory of my life.

I dropped cardio entirely and started lifting weights at my local gym. Within a month, I had lost five pounds. But it wasn't just the weight loss that shocked me—there were other dramatic changes too. My body was less inflamed, I was less bloated, and I no longer woke up feeling like I had been hit by a truck overnight.

And it made me wonder, *What else have I been doing wrong?*

I started to question the calories in/calories out theory that my entire weight-loss education was based on. So, I went looking for answers. I pulled out my human metabolism textbook and notes from college. I had loved this class! I remembered it being the aha moment in my studies when everything I had learned in my biology, biochemistry, anatomy, and physiology courses finally came together. I looked at this 600-page textbook that covered how our bodies metabolize protein, fat, carbohydrates, fiber, vitamins, minerals, and electrolytes and how each system in the body communicates throughout the process. It covered the importance of caloric balance, yes, but I now knew—from experience!—that there was clearly more to the story.

For example, there are hormones in the body that control your appetite, and these hormones are turned on and off based not only on *how much food* you eat but also on *what types of food* you eat. This is because the types of food you eat affect your blood sugar levels, the speed at which you digest food, and the signals traveling from your gut to your brain—all of which play a direct role in your appetite regulation.

So, back when I was attempting to subsist on oatmeal, fat-free yogurt, salads, and cardio, it made perfect sense that I would eventually end up on my floor with my face in a jar of peanut butter at 9:00 p.m. Ghrelin, my hunger hormone, skyrocketed, while leptin, my fullness hormone, plummeted to protect my body from starvation while eating these low-calorie foods. My body was screaming, *Feed me!*

NOT ANOTHER DIET

Every year, 45 million people in the United States go on a diet. Dieting is a $73 billion industry that asks us to count, track, eliminate, eat less, and exercise more; yet, depending on the study that you look at, we know that around 90 percent of these diets fail over the long term. But we keep dieting because the immediate weight loss we experience on our first diet creates a positive association in the brain that's difficult to shed. And dietitians—the professionals you've trusted with your body—are learning to promote the same weight-loss strategies that have an abysmal success rate. The global influence of the diet industry is so powerful that it's even infiltrated our education systems.

As I started to study more and more about how our bodies metabolize food, how they burn and store fat, and what drives hunger and satiety, I began to completely change the way I thought about food. And while I was still very much focused on weight loss, I ditched calorie counting and the rules the diet industry told me I must follow. Instead, I focused on discovering which foods kept me satiated, which foods triggered cravings, which foods energized me after a workout, and which foods helped me sleep better at night. I went from asking *How much less can I eat?* to *How much more can I support my own body?* And over the course of the next year, not only did I shed the weight I had gained but I also healed my relationship with food and my body in the process.

Your story may look different from mine, but I'm guessing you picked up this book because you live with one of these three beliefs:

1. I can't stick to anything, diet or otherwise. My willpower sucks!
2. I can stick to a diet and exercise program like glue, but it doesn't matter because nothing works for me. I never lose any weight!
3. I want nothing to do with diets—I know they don't work. But I still feel like crap, and I'm not sure how to change that.

And like peanut-butter-binging me, you may be feeling frustrated by the fact that you can't get the results you want by following the rules of the diet industry. You might feel like a failure. Or that your body is broken. You might be discouraged and ready to give up. And if you work in the health industry like me, you might even be feeling like a fraud.

If this describes you in any way, stay with me. By the end of this book, you will have the tools not only to lose weight but also to never have to go on another diet again.

I've had the honor of witnessing people from various age ranges and backgrounds repair their metabolism, lose weight, and heal their relationship with food. And here's what I can tell you about them: when they made the decision to ditch the diet industry's rules, they—quite literally—changed their lives. Sure, they lost the weight and felt confident in their own skin, but I also watched them

*   stop obsessing over food and wasting time tracking every morsel of food that went into their mouths;
*   get hired for dream jobs they never would have applied for while in their past bodies;

- eliminate polycystic ovary syndrome (PCOS) symptoms and go from an 84-day to a 32-day menstrual cycle;
- put themselves on dating apps—and meet their dream partner;
- go into remission from bulimia and binge-eating disorders;
- take a picture in a swimsuit on vacation for the first time in 25 years;
- reverse diverticulitis, insulin resistance, and prediabetes;
- achieve clearer skin, drop the afternoon energy slump, and eliminate chronic bloating;
- easily get down on the floor to play with their kids.

PAST DIETER PROFILE

When Sarah first came to me, she was done dieting. She had given up and had decided to accept the fact that she would probably just be depressed and obese for the rest of her life. But the "ditching the diet" approach appealed to her, so she decided to give it one last shot. Within a week, Sarah noticed she was feeling better. Her energy increased and thoughts about food decreased, and even though it took her some time to begin to see physical results, she began to feel something she had never felt in her life—confidence. In two years, she went from a size 22 to a size 10. She is now maintaining that weight easily, and more importantly, she has absolutely no fear of gaining the weight back.

You have the power to change your body and your entire life in the process. The key is both learning how your body's metabolism works *and* understanding the starring role your mind plays in all of this.

Just to be clear: this is not a weight-loss blueprint or another diet book in disguise. Instead, it's a road map that will educate and empower you to make decisions about what to eat, how to move, and how to live in a way that supports your body, no matter what season of life you are in.

HOW TO USE THIS BOOK

This book is designed for the seasoned dieter who has the nutrition facts of every food item in the grocery store memorized *and* for the person who is about to learn about macronutrients for the first time. It's for personal trainers, people who have not yet picked up a dumbbell, and everyone in between.

This is also a book that you can use at your own pace. You may decide to upend everything and make over your life in three days after reading this book, or you may decide to start with breakfast. Both options are beautiful and can lead to permanent positive changes in your body and your life. No matter where you are in life, every step you take toward your metabolism makeover will gradually realign your body and restore it back to metabolic health.

In the upcoming chapters, you'll learn everything you need to know about how your body burns and stores fat, how your appetite is regulated, and how gaining a deep understanding of your metabolism and the role your mindset plays in controlling weight is a critical factor for your long-term success.

I've included several sidebars throughout the book to highlight topics you may find interesting, as well as short client stories in hopes that you will see that some of the women and men who have worked with me are no different from you. Some of the names have been changed for privacy, but all the stories are real.

Let's look at a quick overview of what you'll learn.

Chapter 1: The Metabolic Ecosystem

We start with science. In chapter 1, we'll unpack the concept of metabolism and how it affects you. You'll discover the number one reason you've failed every diet you've ever started, why willpower was never the problem, and how dieting eventually caused your metabolism to "break," for lack of a better term. You'll then be introduced to what I call the Metabolic Ecosystem: blood sugar control, muscle, movement, good sleep, stress management, and a healthy gut. These six pillars are the foundation of our metabolic health, and we'll walk through the details of each one in the upcoming chapters so that you can learn how to eat, exercise, move, sleep, manage stress, and take care of your gut—no matter what life looks like in any given season. At the end of the chapter, you'll find a quiz that will help you assess your current metabolic health and serve as a benchmark going forward.

Chapter 2: Manage Your BS (Blood Sugar, That Is!)

This chapter will completely change the way you think about food. It'll teach you how protein, fat, carbs, and fiber are metabolized; which types of foods keep you full and satiated and which ones tend to make you hungry and have more cravings; and how blood sugar management has been the missing piece of the weight-loss equation all along. You'll find a massive "Build Your Own" (BYO) Meal Guide that offers endless ideas for easy blood-sugar-balancing breakfasts, lunches, dinners, and snacks. Chapter 2 also offers guidance in discovering how much food your body needs to restore your metabolic health.

Chapter 3: Muscle Is Money

In chapter 3, you'll discover why strength training is nonnegotiable for prime metabolic health, the types of strength workouts that give you the biggest bang in the shortest amount of time, and how building muscle will accelerate fat loss more effectively than cardio ever could. To sum up, the more muscle you have, the more calories you burn at rest and the more carbohydrates your body is able to tolerate without weight gain. I'll even help you get started on your new workout routine right away with a one-month, research-backed strength-training program.

Chapter 4: Living in Motion

Weight loss is cool, but have you ever thought about having the ability to go from sitting to standing without assistance when you're 90 years old? In chapter 4, you'll discover why moving your body not only supports good metabolic health today but also sets you up for a better quality of life as you age. Most people struggle with their health and weight in their later years due to a lack of mobility (and a lack of muscle!), but once you're through with chapter 4, you will have the power to change that. And for those of you who can't find the time to add in more movement, you'll find a huge list of fun ways to stack movement on top of your other daily habits.

Chapter 5: Sleep Is Your Magic Pill

Chapter 5 will introduce you to a world beyond diet and exercise, where you'll discover (or be reminded of) the critical impact that sleep has on the body's ability to lose weight. This is where the light bulbs will really start to turn on as you realize how tightly integrated this Metabolic Ecosystem really is. You'll learn how your circadian rhythm is the ultimate ruler of sleep and how to hack your circadian rhythm to get more—and better quality—sleep.

Chapter 6: Yes, You Can Manage Your Stress!

In chapter 6, I'm going to push you to reexamine how you are currently managing stress in your life. In order to achieve optimal metabolic health, you must understand how *all* types of stress affect your body's ability to lose weight. You'll walk away with a very manageable game plan to begin to lessen the stress load on your body, beginning with identifying and eliminating the low-hanging-fruit stressors. Then you'll learn how to make your stress bucket bigger by increasing your capacity for stress through strategies like mindset work, journaling, breath work, and meditation.

Chapter 7: Gut Check

You've probably heard that gut health is important and that issues in the gut can cause digestive problems. But what you may not realize is that these issues can wreak havoc on the entire Metabolic Ecosystem by causing chronic inflammation. This chapter will provide you with a game plan to support the trillions of bacteria that play a key role in the communication between the gut, brain, and nervous system, which, in turn, affects both our physiological and psychological health.

Chapter 8: Train Your Brain

By chapter 8, you will have a completely new relationship with your body! At this point, you will have an action plan for forward movement. You might decide to dive into the deep end by simultaneously incorporating changes to the types of foods you eat, how you exercise and move your body, your sleep schedule, and your mental health practices. Or you might decide to start simple with something you know you can sustain, such as meal-prepping lunches for work instead of relying on takeout. Either way, you'll be ready to learn the art of losing weight by reprogramming your mind for change. I'll introduce an exercise that has changed my life and the lives of thousands of my clients and that will train your brain to help you follow through with your new commitment to yourself.

Chapter 9: Pulling It All Together

This final chapter is where we bring the art and science of weight loss together to create magic. I'll give you a simple three-step process that puts you in control of your week, preparing you to troubleshoot anything that would typically derail you. I'll also teach you the Next Best Choice Framework so that you are equipped to handle any situation life throws your way—surprise donuts at the morning meeting, date night with wine on a Wednesday, or a two-week vacation in the Maldives. I'll teach you how to approach what we often look at as Diet

Danger Zones, like weekends, vacations, holidays, and travel, in a way that allows fun and flexibility while keeping you feeling good and on track with your goals. And, yes, we'll cover how alcohol fits into your life too!

YOU CAN'T FAIL AT THIS!

I don't care if you're a vegan, a bartender, a new mom, male, female, in your twenties or sixties; if you have PCOS; or if you're pregnant: this is a biology class, not a diet plan. Anyone can qualify to sign up for a science course because everyone has the right to learn how their body works. The only difference is that this is a class you cannot fail. Learning how to reestablish a relationship with your body will be an ongoing learning experience; we as human beings are always learning and growing into new versions of ourselves.

Let's dive in.

CHAPTER 1

THE METABOLIC ECOSYSTEM

Allow me to introduce you to Alex. She represents a version of almost every person who has ever gone on a diet. She likely reflects some version of *you*. Yes, even *you*, gentlemen. Many of my clients are women because, well, statistically, women are less satisfied with their bodies, more likely to engage in disordered eating behaviors, and more likely to try different diets. Women think about food and their bodies—often in a negative light—*more often* than men do. But that doesn't mean there aren't millions of men who are also struggling with food and their weight, and the science presented in this book is just as applicable to men as it is to women.

So Alex decides she wants to lose weight, and her first move is to go on a diet. She starts with a combination of the usual tactics. She might

- drop calories;
- cut carbs;
- eat less fat;
- eliminate foods like dairy, grains, legumes, meat, animal products, processed foods, or sugar;
- up her gym time;
- increase her workout intensity;
- decrease her eating windows;

- eliminate alcohol;
- clear her social calendar.

In response to these behavioral changes, Alex will see the weight start to come off. This is exciting and encouraging. Less food plus more exercise equals a better body composition, followed by compliments from friends and family and a temporary boost in confidence. As the weight comes off, her brain connects these dieting behaviors with the dopamine hit that occurs from slipping into an old pair of jeans and receiving compliments from her coworkers or even her mother.

But fear around skipping a workout or eating cheesecake—something that had not previously been on her radar every day—starts to creep in. She starts eating smaller meals and occasionally skipping breakfast, calling it "intermittent fasting." Then she starts feeling hungry. She grits her teeth through hunger and cravings, gets "hangry," overeats after dinner, and beats herself up for not having enough willpower.

Alex begins judging herself when she has a cookie. If she's going to screw up by eating a cookie, she might as well have three. Or six. She notices that when she starts to loosen up with her diet and exercise, the weight quickly comes back on. It must be because she's "getting older" (I hear women say this when they're in their twenties) and her metabolism is slowing down. So she doubles down and starts dragging herself out of bed to get to the gym, even when her body is screaming at her to rest.

Over time, Alex's lifestyle ultimately becomes unsustainable and exhausting. And, worst of all, it doesn't allow her to *live*. Following the diet industry's rules has put her in a losing fight against her own body.

WTF IS GOING ON IN THE BODY?

So, what's really going on here? Let's begin with how the body works.

First, the body needs calories in order to run. Calories come from food sources like protein, fat, fiber, and carbs. Metabolism is the process by which your body takes those calories and turns them into energy. It's just another term for how efficiently the body is burning calories. Later, we will break down how the different food sources are metabolized, how each affects our hunger and satiety hormones, how they impact our blood sugar levels, and how hormones play a role in our body's ability to burn fat. Then we can look at how other factors, such as the way we move, exercise, sleep, manage stress, and live our daily lives, have an impact on our metabolism. For now, the point to remember is that nothing will work without the energy from calories.

We often think about calories only as something that controls our weight, but our bodies need calories in order to pump blood, breathe, digest, and keep our organs functioning every day. We also need energy from calories to do everything, from running a 5K to throwing a ball to your dog or high-fiving a friend. Calories are kind of important. And when we severely limit the amount of calories going into the body, the body adapts and starts requiring fewer calories to live.

Alex normally would require 2,000 calories per day to maintain her weight, which is why she initially lost weight when she started restricting her calorie intake by eating 1,400 calories per day. But because she only ate 1,400 calories per day for months, *her body adapted to the lower calorie intake and now only requires 1,400 calories per day to maintain her weight.* Imagine driving a car a distance that requires a full tank of gas on only three-quarters of a tank. You're going to have to either find a shortcut, learn how to be more fuel efficient, or refill your tank at some point. Your body is exactly the same.

Because our bodies fight caloric restriction tooth and nail, they are hardwired against dieting. Yes, you read that correctly. Diets that restrict calories set you up for failure simply because of how your body works—there's no way around it! And the consequences of dieting don't stop there.

This leads to my second point: you can't disconnect the mind from the body. Dieting mentally sets you up for failure when you begin to equate food with weight gain. Another term for this fear is "food anxiety," and when food anxiety takes over the decision-making part of your brain, the result can look like any of the following:

- a preoccupation with food, such as thinking about what you're going to eat for breakfast when getting into bed at night and what you'll have for lunch and dinner during breakfast

- disordered eating patterns, such as restricting then over-eating or having inflexible or irregular eating patterns for the purpose of weight control
- feeling a "lack of control" around certain foods or feelings of distress like guilt, shame, or disgust when thinking about foods you've eaten or the amount consumed
- feeling stress about a food situation that you have limited or no control over, like a wedding, a vacation, a potluck or dinner where you're not able to order your own food, or a visit to friends or family

This also applies to exercise, including feelings of stress and anxiety when you are not able to exercise for a period of time.

Once the correlation between weight loss and restriction or excess occurs, it can be very difficult to undo. It may start out as just a mild shift in thinking that seems harmless. You may even get a high from caloric restriction and the exercise of willpower to change your behaviors. Humans are motivated by pleasure, and if the body's response to restriction is mostly pleasurable (weight loss), you might not associate anxiety around food as something that will be damaging in the long term. Like, maybe it's good that you fear french fries—you shouldn't be eating them anyway, right?

The vicious cycle of stressing out about food; overeating and undereating; having periods of low-carb, low-fat, or low-protein intake; and chronic overexercising, overcaffeinating, and fasting eventually leads to one destructive destination: a wrecked metabolism.

MISERY AND METABOLIC ISSUES

In the end, all diets lead to some form of metabolic issue. This could look like weight gain, weight-loss resistance, fatigue, anxiety, depression, hair loss, digestive issues, premenstrual syndrome, a dysregulated menstrual cycle, insulin resistance, PCOS, low sex drive, or feeling cold all the time. And I'll get into exactly how and why this happens in chapter 6.

You may be experiencing these issues because you were handed a roll of duct tape (a set of dieting rules) and expected to build a house (lose weight). Not exactly the best building materials, right? Not only were you set up to never be able to finish the project, what you were able to construct is a fragile environment that will eventually break.

You've put so much pressure on yourself to succeed at weight loss, but you've never possessed the right tools to get the job done, *because no one gave them to you.*

Let's check back with Alex. Three years later, the diet she had started just to drop a few unwanted pounds has left her feeling fatigued, bloated, anxious around food, and critical of her body. And if she's like more than 90 percent of dieters, she's at the same weight she was three years ago, if not more.

I bet you identify with at least part, if not all, of Alex's story, because Alex is an amalgamation of three types of clients I see in my programs:

1. The person who believes they *can't stick to anything* because of their past track record or because they have no willpower. They know they can't lose weight and often feel like a failure.
2. The person who does *everything right* and can stick to a diet and exercise program like glue, but *nothing works.* They can't remember the last time they weren't actively trying to lose weight.
3. The person who *just wants to feel good for once* but who is overwhelmed with all the information out there and just wants to know what will work for *their* body. Although they don't identify as a dieter, they're a victim of the diet mentality by proxy and are concerned about following a path that will lead to optimal health and long-term results.

Which type are you? Are you one primary type? Or a combination of two? Or maybe you've been all three at some point in your life? Regardless of your type, you're reading this book because you know intuitively that dieting doesn't work.

It has taught you to be at war with your body.

It has told you that you can't trust yourself to make decisions about food.

It has tricked you into believing that you have no self-control.

Alex, through no fault of her own, believed the diet industry's promise that if she ate less and exercised more, she'd get the physical results she desired. And she did get those physical results—but only temporarily. When Alex's brain connected results with restriction, her mental health was affected. The food anxiety started to creep in. Her thoughts around food became obsessive. Eventually, yo-yo dieting took a toll on her biological health, manifesting in misery and metabolic issues.

Alex's weight-loss journey looked something like this:

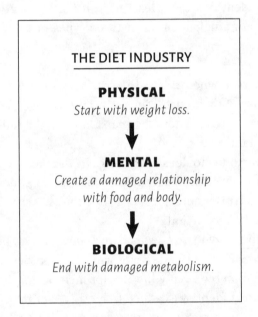

If Alex had flipped this model around, her weight-loss journey would have looked *much* different:

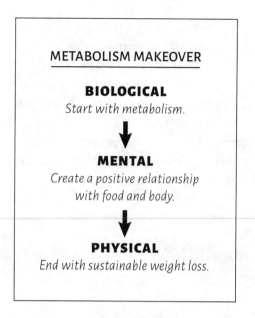

Let's take a deeper look at how having this knowledge would have changed Alex's story.

Meet Alex 2.0

Alex 2.0 wants to lose weight, but she knows that traditional dieting hasn't worked in the past. So she decides to take her weight—and her fate—into her own hands.

She begins with a biological approach by studying how the body actually burns and stores fat. She discovers how protein, fat, carbs, and fiber are metabolized and how each of them plays a role in satiety, hunger, energy, fat burning, and fat storage. She learns about blood sugar—how to manage it and its effect on weight loss. She finds out that weight loss isn't just about a calorie deficit but also about a well-functioning metabolism.

Alex 2.0 feels empowered with all this knowledge. It was quick and easy to get up to speed on how her body works! She doesn't feel like she has to follow a "plan"—she can simply use what she's learned to navigate decisions around food and her body. That knowledge gives her confidence to make choices that are rooted in reason and make sense for her goals. She now knows that there is no longer a wrong choice. She can't "fail" at making empowered decisions for herself. It's not intuitive eating; it's *informed* intuitive eating.

Understanding how her body works has flipped her mental script about food, and she feels ready to walk into any situation—happy hour, vacation, the weekend—feeling confident and empowered instead of anxious and overwhelmed. This approach to weight loss not only is sustainable but also breeds consistency. And sustainability plus consistency equals physical results that last.

DOES INTUITIVE EATING WORK?

The National Eating Disorders Association calls *intuitive eating* a way to make food choices that feel good, without judging yourself or considering the influence of diet culture. While I fully endorse giving the finger to diet culture, I've noticed that clients who have a habit of dieting or restricting don't always know what feels good, because they've been disconnected from their bodies for so long. When you're disconnected from your body, it's hard to know whether the decision to eat a Snickers bar stems from a craving, a blood sugar imbalance, or a decision that truly feels right.

Based on my research and experience, I recommend *informed intuitive eating* instead. This just means that you're starting with a knowledge of human metabolism so that you can make informed decisions about how you want to fuel your body every day.

Your body probably never "needs" a Snickers bar, but a craving for a high-sugar, high-calorie food could mean that you didn't refuel properly after a strength-training workout, you skipped breakfast, or cortisol is pumping through your veins after a high-stakes meeting presentation. With the knowledge you'll learn in this book, you'll know where that craving is coming from, and you'll be able to decide if it's the right choice for you to indulge in that moment. (Maybe you just really love Snickers bars and decide to enjoy one from time to time, and you'll know if that's the case too!)

You'll find, usually fairly quickly, that your body speaks when you listen. I recently had a client laugh when I said her body would start to tell her what it needed: "My body? My body only knows what it *wants*, not what it needs." Within two weeks, she was out running errands and suddenly thought to herself, *I really need some carbs.* She was floored. Based on what she understood about carbohydrates' role in the body, and consistently incorporating them appropriately for her needs over the previous two weeks, she knew exactly what her body needed in that moment.

If Alex 2.0 is faced with the decision of whether to eat a donut for breakfast at the office, she can make that decision from a place of power and strength, not right or wrong. She doesn't black out and spiral out of control if she decides to have the donut; she just eats the donut and then moves on with the rest of her day.

Alex 2.0 never binges or restricts anymore, because eating is no big deal. She feels great every day, so why would she diet? Over time (and with consistency), the weight comes off. It's easy to keep it off, and she approaches maintenance in the same way she approached weight loss.

This is where things get really fun, because when you know how your body works, you can tune in and interpret the signals it's sending you: *Am I hungry? Am I tired? Is this a craving? Do I need more carbs?* You are in control.

The Answer Is in the "Why"

When I started my practice, every client I worked with—whether they were 24 or 64—understood the role of nutrition and exercise in the weight-loss equation; yet, none of them had a grasp on how their metabolism functioned as a whole.

With each diet, they had been given a list of foods to eat or avoid or numbers to shoot for each day. They had been taught how to drive the car but were never given an owner's manual. So, when a warning light went on, they didn't know what it meant or what to do next. They just kept driving until they eventually broke down—and called me.

What I discovered was that they didn't need to learn "how" (the physical aspect of weight loss); they needed to learn "why" (the biological aspect).

Most humans need a "why." *Why* shouldn't I eat a donut every morning for breakfast? "Because I said so" doesn't work on an adult like it does on a six-year-old. (To be honest, does this really even work on a six-year-old?!)

Once my clients began to understand the inner workings of their metabolism (their biology), a switch was flipped in their brains (here come the mental changes). They realized they didn't have to be "good" all week so that they could have the flexibility to enjoy their lives on the weekends. They could always enjoy their lives. It was no longer an all-or-nothing situation—there was an in-between place where they could both feel good and be consistent. While the weight loss wasn't always immediate, the pounds always came off over time (the physical results!), despite most clients claiming they "eat more than ever."

Weight-loss failure is not a physical problem. Focusing on reducing the number on the scale or whittling away the fat in your midsection is exactly where you—and every diet you've ever done—have gone wrong. The true root of weight-loss resistance resides in your mind and your biology. The good news? You have the power to change both.

THE SIX PILLARS

These clients—through no fault of their own—didn't understand that diet and exercise were just a portion of what I call the Metabolic Ecosystem.

The Metabolic Ecosystem is built on six key pillars that create the foundation for your metabolic health. This is your golden ticket not just for losing weight but also for keeping it off for good:

1. **Blood sugar control:** The sugar found in our blood
   comes from the food we eat, and it is our body's primary

source of energy. Blood sugar control is our body's ability to maintain blood sugar levels within a normal range. Uncontrolled blood sugar levels lead to increased cravings and hunger, weight gain, insulin resistance, type 2 diabetes, hormonal imbalances, mood swings, irritability, fatigue, inflammation, and more.

2. **Muscle:** Muscle is our body's most significant site of carbohydrate metabolism, and it has a direct impact on how many calories we burn each day. Strength training will change your body composition by adding visible muscle to your frame and burning more fat.

3. **Movement:** Not to be confused with "exercise," movement is living in motion. Walking, hiking, standing versus sitting, mobility work, stretching—the type and frequency of movement you do daily not only affect your metabolic health today but also will determine how you move—and live—as you age.

4. **Good sleep:** Quality sleep is critical to our bodies' physiological and psychological repair process. Our cognitive function, emotional regulation, stress response, behavior, and appetite during the day are all driven by how we sleep at night.

5. **Stress management:** Stress hormones suppress everything, from your digestive system to your metabolism to your immune function. When we're overexposed to stress, the natural rhythm of the body is disrupted, which can lead to an endless number of health issues, such as weight-loss resistance, chronic inflammation, and digestive problems.

6. **A healthy gut:** Your digestive system is inhabited by trillions of microorganisms, also known as the gut microbiome. The gut microbiome regulates many physiological and psychological functions, from your skin to your heart to your mental well-being to your digestion.

These pillars are not independent variables. This is an interconnected system, with each pillar dependent on the others to varying degrees. If just one pillar is being neglected, it can have a domino effect on the rest of the ecosystem. Here are a few examples of what I mean:

- Sleep affects your blood sugar levels, hunger and satiety hormones, stress response, microbiome, ability to recover from a workout, and energy levels.
- Muscle affects the amount of carbohydrates the body is able to metabolize at once and how many calories are burned at rest.
- Movement and exercise will affect your quality of sleep, as well as the way you manage stress.
- Overexercising can lead to digestive distress and will contribute to your body's stress load.
- The way you manage stress affects the quality and duration of your sleep, the balance in your gut bacteria, how much belly fat you have, and a cascade of hormonal responses in the body that affect metabolism, feelings of hunger and satiety, insulin response, and energy levels.

Before you panic—because maybe you're a new parent not getting enough sleep or you have an injury and can't exercise—don't! This system is intended to be empowering, not limiting. You will have so many more opportunities to fire up your metabolism and take care of your body beyond just diet and exercise. And as with most things in life, you can apply the 80/20 rule—meaning, when you're getting 80 percent of this ecosystem right, you can give yourself grace in the other 20 percent when needed.

Now, this isn't permission to just say, *Well, screw sleep!* But it is encouragement to not throw in the towel, shout *Fuck it all*, and spiral out of control when you pull a muscle and have to stay out of the gym for three weeks. Put that in your 20 percent and stay focused on the other five pillars during that time.

PAST DIETER PROFILE

Here are a handful of examples of how you can use the Metabolic Ecosystem in your favor, no matter what season of life you're currently in:

- Megan is a single mom who's writing a book, parenting her daughter, and running a business that's scaling up (yep, this is me). Because she has a lot on her plate, she is using a meal delivery service to make sure there are blood-sugar-balancing meals readily available. This way she has the extra time and energy to get in workouts and get to bed on time.
- Leon is a night-shift nurse. He pays really close attention to his blood sugar by bringing his own food to work, and he prioritizes eating at regular intervals. He knows he doesn't have as much flexibility in his diet or with his stress levels because the amount (and quality) of sleep he gets is variable, and it's always in that "20 percent I can't change" bucket.
- Camille is postpartum and is living the trifecta of poor sleep, high stress, and no gym time. But she knows how to manage her blood sugar, she sneaks in as many walks as she can, and she's very serious about incorporating stress-relieving practices every day (more on this in chapter 6).
- Bennett has a high-stress accounting job and works 12-hour days. He prioritizes meal prepping on Sunday and eats the same breakfast and lunch every week to keep it simple. He also blocks 30 minutes in his calendar every afternoon to squeeze in a home workout, takes walking phone calls, and has eliminated alcohol during the week, to reduce the stress on his body and to get better sleep.

It may be obvious which areas you're struggling with, or it may not be obvious at all. So I've created a quiz to help you gauge which parts of the Metabolic Ecosystem are slipping into the 20 percent. From there, you decide if you are going to work on bringing those pillars back into the 80 percent or if you need to double down on the pillars that you have more control over in your current season of life.

For example, if sleep is your primary issue but you are taking care of a terminally ill family member, this may not be the time to work on getting a solid eight every night. You may choose instead to ensure you're focused on doing your best with blood sugar control, maintaining muscle, moving your body as much as possible, removing the stressors you have control over, and gut health.

METABOLIC ECOSYSTEM QUIZ

This quiz will be really helpful for you as you begin to develop a new understanding of your body; over time, you'll be so in tune that when one element of the ecosystem is flagging, you'll remember that you have five more pillars to fall back on. You don't have to be perfect every day of your life to wake up looking and feeling fabulous.

As you go through the quiz, you may be tempted to skip ahead to gather the tools you need to raise your score. Don't! Understanding each pillar of the Metabolic Ecosystem thoroughly is key to setting yourself up for lifelong weight loss. No one will have a perfect score, especially the first time you take the quiz. The answers are solely for awareness; that way, you'll know where to focus your energy as you start applying what you learn in the upcoming chapters.

So let's look at this entire ecosystem and determine where you need some help. For each question, write down the letter that corresponds most closely to your answer. Each pillar will be scored separately at the end so you can gauge which pillars need the most attention now. Retake the quiz once a month to keep track of your wins in each section and also to bring awareness to pillars that are lagging.

Pillar 1: Blood Sugar Control

1. When it comes to eating healthy fat (e.g., olive oil, avocado, nuts):
   a. I try to avoid adding fat to my meals.
   b. I eat low fat, but I still add a small amount, like 1 teaspoon of oil or butter, to my meals.
   c. I don't intentionally add fat, but I don't try to eat low fat either.
   d. I make sure to have at least one serving of healthy fat at each meal.

2. When I eat starchy carbohydrates like pasta, potatoes, or rice:
   a. I eat more than 2 cups per meal.
   b. I eat 1.5–2 cups per meal.
   c. I eat 1–1.5 cups per meal.
   d. I eat 1 cup or less per meal.

3. I'm able to stay full and satisfied after a meal:
   a. For 2 hours or less.
   b. For about 3 hours.
   c. It depends on the meal; it could be 2, 3, or 4+ hours.
   d. For about 4 hours.

4. When mealtime is approaching:
   a. I almost always feel irritable (hangry).
   b. I feel hangry often—typically at one meal per day.
   c. I sometimes get hangry, but not every day.
   d. I generally feel calm instead of irritable.

5. I crave high-carbohydrate and high-sugar foods:
   a. At least once per day.
   b. A few times per week.
   c. Once per week.
   d. Once per month or less.

Pillar 2: Muscle

1. I strength train:
   a. Never.
   b. Less than 2 times per week.
   c. 2 or 3 times per week.
   d. 3 or more times per week.

2. My strength workouts look like:
   a. Nothing—I don't strength train.
   b. Random workouts—I'm not following a specific program.
   c. I am consistently going up in weight or reps each week when I work out, and I just started a program like this in the last 3 months.
   d. I am consistently going up in weight or reps each week when I work out, and I've been working out this way for 3+ months.

3. The type of resistance I use when I'm strength training is:
   a. Nothing—I don't strength train.
   b. Light resistance—I don't often reach muscle failure, but if I do, it takes 15+ reps.
   c. Mostly light and medium resistance—to reach muscle failure, it takes 10 or more reps.
   d. A mixture of medium and heavy resistance—to reach muscle failure, it takes 6–8 reps.

4. I do moderate- to high-intensity cardio training like running or cycling:
   a. More than 200 minutes per week.
   b. 150–200 minutes per week.
   c. 100–150 minutes per week.
   d. Less than 100 minutes per week.

5. I eat 30+ grams of protein per meal (e.g., 4–5 ounces of chicken, beef, or fish):
   a. Rarely—I don't eat much protein.
   b. A few times a week.

    c.   Once per day.
    d.   At almost every meal.

Pillar 3: Movement

1.   I get at least 6,000 steps per day (about 3 miles):
    a.   Less than 1 time per week.
    b.   1 or 2 times per week.
    c.   3–5 times per week.
    d.   6+ times per week.

2.   The movement in my daily routine (e.g., job) looks like:
    a.   I sit or stand, in the same position, for 8+ hours per day on most days.
    b.   I make a point to move around and get my blood flowing a few times per day, and/or I split my time between sitting and standing at my desk.
    c.   I take walking meetings, set my alarm to move every hour, and am always thinking of ways I can sneak in more movement.
    d.   I'm moving all day long.

3.   I stretch or work on my mobility:
    a.   Almost never.
    b.   A few times per month.
    c.   At least 2 times per week.
    d.   Almost daily.

4.   When I watch TV:
    a.   I sit or lie down on the couch.
    b.   I sit on the floor.
    c.   I incorporate yoga moves or squats or some other type of dynamic movement.
    d.   I don't watch TV—I'm usually doing something more active instead.

5. I consistently make time for walking, biking, swimming, or another similar activity at a brisk pace but where I can still hold a conversation:
   a. 0–50 minutes per week.
   b. 50–100 minutes per week.
   c. 100–150 minutes per week.
   d. 150 or more minutes per week.

Pillar 4: Good Sleep

1. I feel rested after a night of sleep:
   a. Rarely—I suffer from insomnia regularly.
   b. 1 or 2 nights per week.
   c. 3–5 nights per week.
   d. 6 or 7 nights per week.

2. On average, the amount of sleep I get most nights is (this is actual sleep—not time in bed):
   a. Less than 6 hours per night.
   b. 6–6.5 hours per night.
   c. 6.5–7 hours per night.
   d. 7+ hours per night.

3. I am consistently able to fall asleep within 15 minutes of getting in bed:
   a. 0 or 1 night per week.
   b. 2 or 3 nights per week.
   c. 4 or 5 nights per week.
   d. 6 or 7 nights per week.

4. To my knowledge, I snore:
   a. Almost every night.
   b. At least twice per week, and it may or may not be alcohol related.
   c. Only if I'm congested or drink alcohol.
   d. Never, that I'm aware of.

5. When I wake up in the middle of the night, it takes me longer than 15 minutes to fall back asleep:
   a. 6 or 7 nights per week.
   b. 3–5 nights per week.
   c. 1 or 2 nights per week.
   d. It rarely takes me longer than 15 minutes to fall back asleep.

Pillar 5: Stress Management

1. I feel very stressed:
   a. Almost 75–100 percent of the time—I feel like I can't take it much longer.
   b. 50–75 percent of the time—it affects my quality of life.
   c. 25–50 percent of the time—it affects my quality of life sometimes, but for the most part, I manage it well.
   d. Less than 25 percent of the time—stress rarely affects my quality of life.

2. Preventive stress management, like journaling, meditation, or breath work, is something:
   a. I rarely do.
   b. I do, but I'm not consistent about it.
   c. I do a few times per week.
   d. I practice daily.

3. The number of rest days from workouts that I take each week are:
   a. Typically 0—no days off.
   b. 1 day, but it's usually active rest like a hike or yoga class.
   c. 1 day.
   d. 2+ days.

4. I do high-intensity interval training, take boot-camp-style workout classes, and/or run for 60+ minutes:
   a. 5+ days per week.
   b. 3 or 4 days per week.

    c.   1 or 2 days per week.

    d.   It's rare that I do these types of workouts.

5.   I avoid eating starchy carbohydrates (e.g., pasta, rice, bread, fruit, beans, potatoes):

    a.   Almost always—I eat a strict ketogenic, carnivore, or very low-carb diet.

    b.   Most days—I do include them on weekends or special occasions.

    c.   3–5 days per week—I carb cycle.

    d.   I don't avoid them—I eat at least one type of starchy carb every day.

Pillar 6: A Healthy Gut

1.   I experience digestive issues like bloating, constipation, diarrhea, or upset stomach:

    a.   Nearly every day.

    b.   At least once or twice a week.

    c.   If I eat a certain food, but for the most part, my digestion is fine.

    d.   Almost never.

2.   When it comes to food intolerance or sensitivities:

    a.   I'm intolerant or sensitive to several foods; my diet is very limited because most foods bother me.

    b.   I'm intolerant or sensitive to at least one food, but I'm still able to eat a variety of foods.

    c.   I'm not sure if I'm intolerant or sensitive to any foods.

    d.   I'm not intolerant or sensitive to any foods.

3.   I experience heartburn/acid reflux:

    a.   Almost daily.

    b.   Often enough that it's a problem in my life.

    c.   On occasion, if I eat a certain food or drink alcohol before going to bed.

    d.   Almost never.

4. When it comes to having consistent skin conditions like acne, psoriasis, eczema, and/or recurring rashes (if you're on medication, including birth control, to manage skin issues, please answer this question as if you were not taking the medication):
    a. I have 3 or more.
    b. I have 2.
    c. I have 1.
    d. I don't have any.

5. I take antibiotics:
    a. At least once per year, and/or there was a time in my life when I took a long, heavy dose for a particular reason.
    b. About every 2 years.
    c. About every 5 years.
    d. Rarely—less than 3 times in my life.

Bonus: *Your Relationship with Food and Your Body*

1. When I have a craving:
    a. I use my willpower to fight it, and it often causes me a lot of stress.
    b. Sometimes I can calmly decide if I want the food at that particular moment or not and move on; sometimes I'm using my willpower to fight it.
    c. I'm usually able to calmly decide if I want the food at that particular moment or not and move on, but I do have certain foods I struggle with.
    d. It's no big deal; I decide if I want the food at that particular moment or not and move on.

2. My relationship with food looks like this:
    a. Food is the enemy, and I think about it 24/7.
    b. It depends on the day, but I have more bad feelings about food than good.
    c. It depends on the day, but I have more good feelings about food than bad.
    d. Food is fuel, and I rarely think about it.

3. My relationship with my body looks like this:
    a. Not many days go by where I don't have negative thoughts
        about how I look or feel.
    b. I have some love and respect for what my body has done for
        me, but most days I still think negatively about it.
    c. I have love and respect for what my body has done for me,
        but occasionally I have negative thoughts toward it.
    d. I love my body.

4. When it comes to my appetite:
    a. I often eat when not hungry just because food is in front of
        me. I have a hard time quitting eating certain foods even
        when I'm full.
    b. I eat when not hungry just because food is in front of me
        about 50 percent of the time. I have a hard time quitting eat-
        ing certain foods even when I'm full about 50 percent of the
        time. It just depends on the day and how I'm feeling.
    c. I typically eat when I'm hungry and quit when I'm satisfied,
        but there are certain foods I struggle with.
    d. I almost always eat when I'm hungry and quit when I'm satis-
        fied.

5. When I'm in a food situation where I'm not entirely in control of
    the menu:
    a. I stress out and even cancel plans so that I don't have to be
        around "off-limit" foods.
    b. I stress out, but it's not so extreme that I'll cancel plans or
        spiral out of control over it.
    c. I will have some anxiety, but I manage it.
    d. I'm fine with it—*food* and *stress* are not two words that go
        together in my vocabulary.

Score your answers:

A = 1 point

B = 2 points

C = 3 points

D = 4 points

Total your scores in each section. For example, if you selected answers a, c, b, a, and d in the "Blood Sugar Control" section, your total score in that section would be

$$1 + 3 + 2 + 1 + 4 = 11.$$

If you scored between 15 and 20, you likely don't currently struggle with that pillar. Use the corresponding chapters to learn more about what makes these pillars so important to continue to take care of and to pick up some additional tools to try out.

If you scored between 10 and 15, you should be able to find some quick wins by implementing some of the tools found in the following chapters.

If you scored between 5 and 10, make a mental note that that pillar needs more attention. Did you score between 5 and 10 in every section? Great! You are in the right place, and I can't wait to support you throughout this book. These numbers simply illustrate where you are on your unique path, and meeting your metabolism where it's at will be an ongoing process. This is not a race but a journey to feeling good in your body again.

Note that while "Your Relationship with Food and Your Body" is not an official element of the Metabolic Ecosystem, it is an essential part of this process. This relationship is vital to understand if you want to lose weight *and* keep it off, and it directly affects the choices you make around the Metabolic Ecosystem every day. You'll find this theme woven throughout the book.

30-SECOND SUMMARY

1. Diets that focus on calorie restriction *mentally* set you up for failure. The more you restrict, the more you have obsessive thoughts about food, and the more likely you are to fall into "all-or-nothing thinking," which can lead to cycles of binging and restricting.

2. Diets that focus on calorie restriction also *biologically* set you up for failure. The body needs a certain number of calories to function optimally, so when we deprive the body of the calories it needs to run, the body will do whatever it takes to make sure it has what it needs. This can vary from increased hunger, which can often lead to overeating, to a lowered metabolic rate, which can lead to weight-loss resistance.

3. The Metabolic Ecosystem consists of six key pillars that create the foundation for your metabolic health: blood sugar control, muscle, movement, good sleep, stress management, and a healthy gut. Understanding and utilizing this ecosystem is your golden ticket not just for losing weight but also for keeping it off for good. And while all six pillars are equally important, learning how to manage your BS (blood sugar) can change the way you feel and start to reshape your relationship with food almost immediately and will give you momentum for moving through the remaining pillars.

CHAPTER 2

MANAGE YOUR BS
(BLOOD SUGAR, THAT IS!)

Food is a necessary element of life; we already covered that when talking about calories in chapter 1. Eating is something we need to do so frequently that it can sometimes seem like a hassle when we're just trying to check things off the never-ending to-do list. So we turn to quicker and easier options without putting much thought into what's going into our bodies. Or maybe we do have an inkling—everyone knows that fast food isn't a great option—but we feel that we don't have a choice or just value the time saved more than the quality of that fuel. But what if you didn't always have to choose between your time and the quality of your meals?

This chapter will seriously change the way you look at food, and that's why we're talking about it first. If you can learn to manage your BS (blood sugar), you will calm your raging appetite, crush cravings, have steady energy all day, and keep your body burning fat even while you sleep.

WHAT IS BLOOD SUGAR AND WHY DO WE CARE?

Put simply, blood sugar is the amount of glucose (sugar) in the blood. But before we go any further into what that means, we have to talk about the dirtiest word in dieting right now—*carbohydrates*—and its impact on blood sugar.

Carbohydrates are one of three types of macronutrients found in food and drinks. Macronutrients are essential nutrients that our bodies need to function. The other two macronutrients, which we will cover later in the chapter, are protein and fat. Sugar, starches, and fiber are all classified as different types of carbohydrates.

Sugar is a simple carbohydrate that the body quickly absorbs because it's already in a form that can be immediately utilized for energy. There are naturally occurring sugars in foods like milk and fruit, although most sugar we come across is added to foods like candy, ice cream, juices, dressings, condiments, and cereals. It is estimated that up to 60 percent of the foods you find in the grocery store contain added sugar.

Starches, or starchy carbs, are the most common type of carbohydrate and are also referred to as complex carbs. Starchy carbs are made up of sugar molecules that are strung together in a chain, so the body has to first break them down into sugar in order to utilize them. Although starchy carbs eventually turn into sugar in the body, they take a little longer to break down and provide longer-lasting energy than eating straight sugar. Starchy carbs include foods like potatoes, rice, beans, grains, and fruit.

Once carbohydrates are broken down into sugar, the sugar enters the bloodstream—hence, the term *blood sugar*. Next, the pancreas is triggered to release the storage hormone insulin, which picks up the sugar and delivers it to muscle, liver, and fat cells to be either used immediately or stored for later. So, both starchy carbs and sugar raise blood sugar levels as they are broken down and metabolized in the body. High blood sugar spikes that are due to large amounts of consumed carbohydrates trigger a rush of insulin into the bloodstream. This is significant for two reasons:

1. When you constantly hit your body with more carbohydrates than it can handle at once, you'll experience chronically elevated insulin levels, which, over time, can lead to insulin resistance, heightened blood sugar, and even type 2 diabetes.

2. Large amounts of insulin in the bloodstream block the
    body from burning fat.

Remember Alex from chapter 1? We walked through a similar sce-
nario with her, but let's review how blood sugar behaves when we eat a
so-called healthy açaí bowl:

1. For breakfast, you choose an açaí bowl made with açaí,
    banana, honey, strawberries, granola, and coconut. Most
    of these foods are made up of carbohydrates, though
    coconut contains some fat. Your açaí bowl contains 360
    calories, 5 grams of fat, 75 grams of carbohydrates, 31
    grams of sugar, 1 gram of fiber, and 4 grams of protein.
2. As your body begins to digest the açaí bowl, your blood
    sugar rises quickly as carbohydrates are converted into
    sugar.
3. The pancreas releases insulin to mop up all the sugar (at
    this point, we will use the scientific term *glucose*) in the
    bloodstream. It is first dropped into muscle and liver
    cells, as these cells are where energy from carbohydrates
    is stored. Once those stores are full, the leftover glucose
    is stored in fat cells. Yes, even your fancy açaí bowl will be
    stored as fat if it has nowhere else to go.
4. As insulin stuffs excess glucose into cells, our blood sugar
    levels start to crash. The crash makes us feel tired, groggy,
    and hungry . . . already! You just ate two hours ago, and
    you're starting to feel a grumble in your stomach.
5. Often after a blood sugar crash, we'll reach for *anything*
    to feel normal again. An apple? A Perfect Bar? A vanilla
    latte? A handful of M&M's? All of these will cause blood
    sugar to spike right back up. And then we start the cycle
    over again.

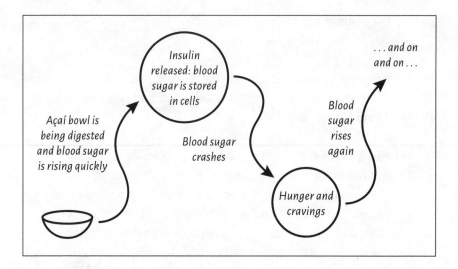

To recap, blood sugar goes up; insulin is released; glucose is shuffled into the muscle, liver, and fat cells; blood sugar levels drop; we start to feel lethargic; our brain tells us we need more sugar; and we dive headfirst into the carbs again.

Wait, does this mean I can't have my $16 bowl of açaí for breakfast anymore?

You can have your açaí, but just know that even nutrient-rich foods like bananas, strawberries, and açaí are made up of primarily carbohydrates and can wreak havoc on your blood sugar when eaten in large amounts. This can lead to high insulin levels, fat storage, blood sugar crashes, and cravings throughout the day. The solution is learning how to tame your blood sugar without giving up carbs.

Keeping blood sugar levels under control prevents the body from storing fat. This gives you a lot of power at mealtime, because it takes away the idea that you have to deprive yourself of calories and, instead, creates the freedom to choose foods that will keep your blood sugar steady.

BALANCE YOUR BLOOD SUGAR WITH PHFF

In order to keep your blood sugar in check, I want you to remember this simple acronym: *PHFF*—for *protein, healthy fat,* and *fiber.*

That's it. That's the chapter. I could just give you a list of approved proteins, healthy fats, and fiber-containing foods; tell you to eat them at every meal; and call it a day.

But I won't do that, because I can't just tell you what to eat! That would make this just like every other diet you've tried in the past. You've gotta learn exactly how protein, healthy fat, and fiber affect your blood sugar levels so that you can go out into the wild and be empowered to make your own decisions.

Protein, healthy fat, and fiber are powerful agents in blood sugar control and satiety. Each has its own specific, rock-star function, which is why it's important to incorporate all three—or at *least* two out of the three—at every meal. And what's cool about eating PHFF is that, instead of taking 10 precious minutes to tally up calories, carbs, fat, and protein when you're on a diet, all you'll have to do is run through a quick checklist:

Where's my protein? Healthy fat? Fiber?

And you can do this with anything; PHFF isn't limited to meal prep. Understanding how these three nutrients work in your body— along with carbs—is knowledge you can take with you on vacation, on road trips, and out to happy hours.

PHFF can look like a simple breakfast of eggs, broccoli, and avocado for breakfast, or it can look like a wild Friday night with a bun-less cheeseburger, fries, and a martini. The beauty of this simple structure is that there's wiggle room to enjoy food. And when you enjoy what you're eating, there's no reason to panic every time you leave your house to eat. Let's break down these three macronutrients and what makes them so beneficial for our bodies.

Protein

Protein is a macronutrient made up of 20 different amino acids, which are the building blocks for our muscles, bones, skin, hair, nails, and cartilage. Protein also plays an important role in the creation and maintenance of every cell and enzyme in our body.

Protein-rich foods include animal products like beef, chicken, seafood, pork, eggs, and dairy products. Plant-based foods like beans, lentils, nuts, seeds, and tofu are less protein dense but serve as protein sources as well.

Protein is your key macronutrient when it comes to keeping you full, revving up your metabolism, and getting you lean. It's a natural appetite suppressant that has the added bonus of maintaining precious muscle tissue. You may not always have to eat a lot of protein to lose weight, but it's going to make your life a hell of a lot easier, and results will come a hell of a lot more quickly! There are three facts about protein intake you can use to your advantage for weight loss:

1. Protein lends to muscle synthesis and maintenance, which in turn boosts your metabolic rate; more on this in chapter 3.
2. Protein has the highest thermal effect of food (TEF), which means, when consumed, protein increases your metabolic rate more than carbohydrates and fat do.
3. Protein is the most satiating macronutrient, which means, when compared gram for gram with carbohydrates and fat, protein keeps you fullest.

How Much Protein Do I Need?

While I want you to ditch the rules of the diet industry, the reality is that our bodies have some inherent needs in terms of how much protein (in combination with the other macronutrients!) it requires in order to look, feel, and function optimally. So, let's walk through my recommendations, which are based on both research and clinical experience. I want you to look at these recommendations as bumpers, not rules. My three main goals in giving you these parameters are to help you begin to heal your metabolism, feel your best, and give you the information you need to make optimal decisions for your own body.

The US Department of Agriculture's recommended dietary allowance is 0.36 grams of protein per pound of body weight. This would mean that if you are 160 pounds, you would need about 58 grams of protein per day. But 0.36 grams of protein per pound of body weight is an absurdly low amount of protein that will only keep you *alive*, not *living* and aging optimally. I do not recommend going this low with your protein, unless you don't like lean muscle or staying satiated (hopefully, that's no one!).

The bodybuilding industry often tells you to shoot for 1 gram of protein per pound of body weight in order to build or maintain muscle. This would mean that if you are 160 pounds, you would need about 160 grams of protein per day. One gram of protein per pound of body weight is great for satiety, which is important during weight loss. But it's not necessary for muscle growth or maintenance and is unrealistic for those with a higher body weight.

My recommendation is based on both science and helping thousands of clients lose weight over the years. The most current research tells us that 0.8 grams of protein per pound of body weight is the sweet spot for building and maintaining muscle. This would mean that if you are 160 pounds, you would need about 128 grams of protein per day.

For many, 0.8 grams of protein per pound of body weight works well, but since protein is not needed to support fat cells, this number can again get really intimidating and can be unnecessary for those who are significantly overweight. So, there are two options when determining your daily protein needs:

0.8 x weight in pounds = total protein per day

or

1 x weight in pounds at a body mass index (BMI) of 25 = total protein per day.

While I believe using BMI as an indicator of health is the biggest joke in medicine, what I'm looking for here is an approximate body weight that will more accurately reflect how much muscle actually needs to be supported. The second formula works really well for those who have a significant amount of weight to lose, because it keeps protein needs on the higher end for satiation, without going completely overboard and creating a plan that is unreasonable to follow.

BMI: HELPFUL METRIC OR ARBITRARY NUMBER?

Two hundred years or so ago, a mathematician in Belgium created a formula to measure obesity—the BMI. It determines one's body mass by using weight, in kilograms, divided by the square of height, in meters. According to the website of the Centers for Disease Control and Prevention, BMI is an easy screening method for weight category—underweight, healthy weight, overweight, and obese. The formula does not account for differences based on sex, race, or age, as the sample population used to create the formula included only "healthy" European men. The formula also does not account for bone, muscle, and fat, all of which make up a human's body weight and are highly variable in weight.

Using BMI as a tool to evaluate a person's metabolic health is easy, but it offers no insight into a person's actual body composition, which is a far more relevant parameter for our health status. Body-fat percentage, amount of visceral fat, bone-mineral density, and lean-muscle mass are more accurate determiners of body composition than one's height and weight.

WEIGHT (IN POUNDS) AT BMI OF 25 (BY HEIGHT)

4' 10"	4' 11"	5'	5' 1"	5 '2"	5' 3"
120	124	128	133	137	142

5' 4"	5' 5"	5' 6"	5' 7"	5' 8"	5' 9"
146	151	155	160	165	170

5' 10"	5' 11"	6'	6' 1"	6' 2"	6' 3"
175	180	185	190	195	200

Now, how do you put these formulas to work? Let's go back to our 160-pound person, and let's say this person is 5' 5". We have two options to determine their protein needs:

Option 1 (based on body weight): 0.8 x 160 = 128 grams of protein.
Option 2 (based on a BMI of 25 for someone 5'5"): 1 x 151 = 151 grams of protein.

Next, choose the lower amount of protein as this person's protein needs, which is 128 grams. Protein is not needed to support fat tissue, which is why we choose the lower amount. If they were eating 128 grams of protein per day and ate three times per day, they would want to shoot for about 43 grams of protein per meal. What if they eat four times per day? Cool. That's 32 grams of protein per meal.

There's no reason to obsess over these numbers. I repeat, there is *no* reason to obsess over these numbers! But knowledge is power and offers you control, which in turn leaves no room for anxiety about eating.

Use the following chart to get an appropriate amount of protein in your meals. Yes, you'll have to do some basic math in the beginning. This is what informed intuitive eating is all about! Sometimes it can be helpful to use a cheap food scale for a few days to see what 5 ounces of steak looks like, because you are likely grossly undereating protein. I still pull mine out from time to time to make sure I'm eating enough. But, remember, we are not striving for perfection. It's not about measuring or calculating to restrict. It's about making sure you are fueling your body with what it needs until it becomes second nature.

Knowing this, it'll start to become really easy to put together meals to hit your protein goals each day—no tracking necessary!

ANIMAL PROTEINS (SERVING SIZE FOR COOKED PROTEIN)

- 1 large egg = 6 g
- 4 oz boneless, skinless chicken breast = 34 g
- 4 oz chicken thighs = 30 g
- 4 oz pork chops = 31 g
- 4 oz 90%-lean ground beef = 30 g
- 4 oz ground turkey = 30 g
- 4 oz ground bison = 29 g
- 4 oz lamb = 28 g
- 4 oz sirloin = 30 g
- 4 oz shrimp = 28 g
- 4 oz wild salmon = 27 g
- 4 oz halibut = 30 g
- 5 oz can of tuna = 30 g
- 4 oz nitrate-free deli turkey = 20 g
- 1/2 cup whole-milk Greek yogurt = 10 g
- 1/2 cup 2% cottage cheese = 14 g
- protein powder (varies—see resources for recommendations)
- collagen powder (varies—see resources for recommendations)

Yes, plant-based protein is protein too! But I've made a separate graphic, since plant-based proteins have less protein density. This means you have to eat a higher quantity of plant-based sources to get the same amount of protein that you'd get from an animal-based source. For example, in order to eat 30 grams of protein from steak, you would have to eat 4 ounces of cooked sirloin, which clocks in at 230 calories. To eat 30 grams of protein from black beans, you would have to eat 2 cups of beans at 450 calories. To eat 30 grams of protein from edamame, you would have to eat 1 1/2 cups of edamame at 300 calories. And one more—to eat 30 grams of protein from peanut butter, you would have to eat almost a 1/2 cup of peanut butter at 735 calories. While we are not focused on calories, it's important to demonstrate how much more food it takes to eat 30 grams of protein when eating plant-based protein versus animal protein. We've proved that counting calories is a poor long-term strategy for weight loss, but the chronic overconsumption of calories *does* lead to weight gain.

These plant-based proteins have more calories and are less satiating per calorie than animal proteins because they generally contain *more* fat or carbs than do animal proteins. For example, 2 cups of black beans have 88 grams of carbs, and a 1/2 cup of peanut butter has 65 grams of fat. Compare that with the 4 ounces of sirloin, which has 0 grams of carbs and 16 grams of fat. Because of this, you may not be able to hit the daily protein goals outlined in this section if you are a strict vegan. My recommendation is to still shoot for at least 100 grams of protein per day by eating the protein-rich plant sources from the following chart and to supplement with a plant-based protein powder once per day.

PLANT-BASED PROTEINS

- 1 cup cooked beans (black, kidney, pinto, etc.) = 15 g
- 1 cup cooked lentils = 18 g
- 1 cup cooked chickpeas = 15 g
- 1 oz nuts = 5–7 g
- 2 tbsp chia seeds = 3 g
- 3 tbsp hemp seeds = 9 g
- 1/4 cup pumpkin seeds = 10 g
- 1/4 cup sunflower seeds = 5 g
- 2 tbsp flaxseed = 5 g
- 1 cup extra-firm tofu = 20 g
- 1 cup edamame (shelled) = 17 g
- 2 tbsp nutritional yeast = 8 g
- 1 cup cooked peas = 9 g
- 2 tbsp spirulina = 8 g
- 1 cup tempeh = 32 g

- 1 cup cooked quinoa = 8 g
- 4 oz seitan = 24 g
- 2 tbsp peanut butter powder = 5 g
- 2 tbsp peanut butter = 8 g
- 2 tbsp almond butter = 7 g

Healthy Fat

Fat is the third and final macronutrient we consume through our diet. There are five kinds of fats, and knowing the different types is important because some fats will support metabolic health while others can be damaging.

If you've been hanging out in diet culture for a long time, you know that fat has gotten a bad rap over the years as something that "makes you fat." But the reality is that *healthy* fat is critical for aiding in the absorption of crucial vitamins like A, D, E, and K; regulating body temperature; supporting the immune system; keeping hormones balanced; and making our food taste good (yes, this is critical!).

But not all fat is created equal. Let's look at common sources of each type and at what exactly is happening in the body when we consume these different fats:

- Saturated fats: This type of fat has had a bad rap for a while, but when we look at the results of long-term studies, the evidence against saturated fat is weak. What's important when consuming saturated fat—as with any fat!—is focusing on whole-food sources like whole-fat dairy, coconut milk, and grass-fed beef. Saturated fats are needed to form cell membranes, transport cholesterol for hormone synthesis and cellular repair, and maintain a healthy gut.
- Monounsaturated fats: Monounsaturated fats are known to improve the markers that indicate the risk of cardiovascular disease and may reduce the incidence of heart disease. They've been shown to improve cholesterol levels

and reduce both blood pressure and inflammation. They are found in olives, avocados, and some nuts.

- Omega-3 fatty acids: These fats, from sources like cold-water fatty fish and some plant foods like walnuts and seeds, decrease the risk of heart disease by 35 percent (a much higher percentage than that for statin therapy!) with only 200–500 milligrams per day. They are all essential for brain development, which is why you'll often find omega-3 fatty acid supplements marketed to improve memory and concentration.
- Omega-6 fatty acids: These fats come from a variety of plant and animal foods but are primarily found in industrially processed oils like canola, vegetable, corn, soybean, rapeseed, and sunflower. They are essential to our survival in small amounts, but we eat these fats in excess because of the amount of oils we consume. The overconsumption of omega-6 fatty acids raises inflammatory metabolites, increasing systemic inflammation in the body.
- Trans fats: There are some naturally occurring trans fats in animal products, but artificial trans fats are found in hydrogenated vegetable oils. For every 2 percent increase in calories from trans fats, the risk of heart disease and type 2 diabetes nearly doubles.

Going forward, when I talk about healthy fat, you can assume I'm talking about saturated, monounsaturated, and omega-3 fatty acids.

When it comes to the first pillar, blood sugar control, healthy fat has a superpower: the ability to slow everything down. As blood sugar starts to rise, fat acts as a buffer to slow the spike and keep blood sugar levels steadier. It also slows digestion, and the slower we digest food, the fuller and more satisfied we'll feel for a longer period of time.

When you feel fuller longer and you don't experience those sharp blood sugar spikes and crashes, then you don't get the signals from your brain that tell your body it needs more sugar or carbs ASAP. Thus, fat is a huge help in curbing those midafternoon or late-night cravings that can end in a peanut butter and Oreo binge.

How Much Fat Do I Need?

The dietary reference intake for fat is 20–35 percent of daily calories. This would equal 47–82 grams of fat per day for someone eating 2,100 calories per day. Less, of course, if you're eating less and more if you're eating more. However, if you want balanced hormones (and happy periods, if you have them), I wouldn't recommend dipping below 25 percent.

I know you're thinking, *What am I supposed to do with that percentage?!* Nothing—it's just a reference point. Instead of using a percentage to determine fat intake, I'm going to teach you how to tune into your internal calorie counters by gauging how long you're able to stay satiated between meals. As long as you're eating as much protein as you're supposed to be eating and you've got some fiber on your plate (more on that soon), how long you can go between meals is an accurate indicator of appropriate fat intake.

If 10 grams of fat equals one serving of fat, shoot for one to three servings (10–30 grams) of fat per meal or one to two servings (10–20 grams) of fat per snack. This parameter works well for most people.

ABOUT 10 g OF HEALTHY FAT

- 1 tbsp nut butter
- 1 oz cheese
- 1/3 avocado
- 2 tsp olive oil
- 2 tsp avocado oil
- 2 tsp coconut oil
- 2 tsp butter made from milk from grass-fed cows
- 2 tsp ghee made from milk from grass-fed cows
- 1/4 cup canned full-fat coconut milk
- 2 tbsp heavy cream
- 2 tbsp seeds (sunflower, sesame, pumpkin, etc.)
- 3 tbsp nuts

Fiber

Fiber is a magical nutrient that stunts the blood sugar response, soaks up toxins in the digestive tract, flips on satiety hormones, feeds the healthy bacteria in your gut, and helps to form nice, solid, all-star poops. Though it is a type of carbohydrate, it behaves much differently than a carbohydrate, so, for our purposes, I'm not going to classify it as one. When we think of carbs, we think of fast energy because they are broken down quickly and absorbed into the bloodstream. Fiber, however, cannot be broken down at all. It moves through the digestive tract unbothered while, quite literally, stretching the stomach lining to trigger the feeling of fullness. Fiber also acts like fat in that it helps to prevent blood sugar spikes.

If you were to sit down two people, one with a bowl of white rice and the other with a bowl of black beans, and instruct them to eat until they were full, my money would be on the person who is eating the beans to get full first. Both foods contain primarily carbohydrates, but only one of those foods contains several grams of fiber (and protein!). Now, if you were to add a bowl of steak to the competition? No contest—steak would be the winner because of the satiating high-protein content.

There are two types of fiber—soluble and insoluble—but for the purposes of this book, we'll lump them together as "fiber." It's pretty easy to incorporate both into your diet, so don't sweat keeping them separate (unless you've been told by your health-care practitioner to avoid one, of course).

Some great sources of fiber are nonstarchy vegetables like broccoli, cauliflower, and asparagus, as well as chia seeds, flaxseed, beans, lentils, nuts, grains, and fruits like berries, apples, and pears.

How Much Fiber Do I Need?

The standard recommendation for fiber intake is 21–25 grams per day for women and 30–38 grams per day for men. To simplify, I like to make a blanket recommendation of 25–35 grams of fiber per day for most people.

Since only 7 percent of Americans are meeting fiber recommendations, I think what's more important than obsessing over the numbers is simply having an awareness that you probably need to be eating more fiber at every meal.

So where does fiber come from? Understanding how much fiber is in the foods you eat is a great place to start building that awareness. I would bet that if I were to ask you what a high-fiber lunch looks like, you might say a big green salad. But look at this:

YOUR AVERAGE SALAD

- 2 cups spinach = 1.5 g fiber
- 1/2 cup chopped cucumber = 0.5 g fiber
- 1/2 cup chopped tomato = 0 g fiber
- 1/2 cup chopped broccoli = 2.5 g fiber

Total: 4.5 g fiber

HIGH-FIBER SALAD

- 1 cup shredded cabbage = 1.5 g fiber
- 1 cup shredded romaine = 1 g fiber
- 1/2 cup shredded carrots = 1 g fiber
- 1/2 cup chopped broccoli = 2.5 g fiber
- 1/2 cup marinated artichoke hearts = 7 g fiber
- 1 tsp chia seeds = 2 g fiber

Total: 15 g fiber

So, with this in mind, let's get into some of my favorite high-fiber foods.

FRUIT FIBER

- 1 apple = 4 g
- 1 avocado = 10 g
- 1 cup blueberries = 4 g
- 1 cup blackberries = 8 g
- 1 cup raspberries = 8 g
- 1 pear = 6 g

NONSTARCHY VEGGIE FIBER

- 1 cup cooked artichoke = 10 g
- 1 cup cooked asparagus = 4 g
- 1 cup cooked broccoli = 5 g
- 1 cup cooked brussels sprouts = 4 g
- 1 cup raw cauliflower = 2 g
- 1 cup cooked collard greens = 8 g
- 1 cup cooked carrots = 4 g
- 1 cup cooked eggplant = 2 g

OTHER FIBER

- 1 tbsp acacia fiber = 6 g
- 1 tbsp chia seeds = 5 g
- 1 tbsp flaxseed = 2 g

- 1 cup cooked black beans = 15 g
- 1 cup cooked kidney beans = 12 g
- 1 cup cooked chickpeas = 13 g
- 1 cup cooked edamame (shelled) = 10 g
- 1 cup cooked peas = 8 g
- 1 cup cooked lentils = 16 g
- 1 cup cooked quinoa = 5 g
- 1 oz almonds = 3.5 g
- 1 oz pistachios = 3 g

A Blood-Sugar-Balancing Açaí Bowl

With this system, you never have to feel like you can't eat something because it's "off-limits" or because it's going to "ruin your progress." PHFF is always the answer to "Can I eat that?"

Now, still feeling salty about that açaí bowl? Let's take a look at how you can apply PHFF to your bowl so that you can enjoy your favorite breakfast *while* keeping your blood sugar steady and your body burning fat:

1. Make sure your açaí is not sweetened. Check the label when buying at the store and look for added sugar, or ask your local açaí bowl shop. It's not a naturally sweet fruit, so it's pretty low in sugar if you're not adding sugar to it.
2. Skip all the additional fruits being blended with the açaí. Blending bananas, pineapple, and mangos into the bowl and also adding more on top makes a sugar bomb.
3. Add a high-quality protein powder that is free of artificial sweeteners, sugar, vegetable oils, and soy.
4. Add fiber—chia seeds, flaxseed, and coconut flakes are some of my personal favorites. Raspberries and blackberries are two of the most high-fiber fruits too.
5. Make sure there is a fat source. This could be coconut milk, coconut flakes, nuts, or nut butter.

For example, an unsweetened açaí bowl blended with raspberries and a scoop of protein powder, topped with chia seeds, coconut flakes, and almond butter, will clock in at around 450 calories, 22 grams of fat, 34 grams of carbs, 10 grams of fiber, and 30 grams of protein. I would be willing to bet this will keep you full until lunch!

SO, WHAT ABOUT CARBS?

Let's do a brief review.

Macronutrients are broken down into glucose in the body, which causes our blood sugar to rise. Consuming protein, healthy fat, and fiber along with starchy carbs can blunt the blood sugar response to keep our blood sugar steady, as well as trigger our satiety hormones.

You may be thinking that, in order to avoid blood sugar spikes, you should avoid carbs altogether, but that *could not be further from the truth.*

Your number one goal for eating carbohydrates is not to avoid them; it's to utilize and store them in the liver and muscle cells (instead of in the fat cells). So how do we make sure that happens? By understanding your carbohydrate threshold.

This is exactly what it sounds like: the amount of carbs your liver and muscle can uptake at each meal. Though the carbohydrate threshold varies from person to person, research shows, on average, that the number is around 30–40 grams of carbs. And when you factor in how many of those carbs we'll use for immediate energy, that threshold jumps to around 50 grams per meal.

But, don't worry, you don't have to know how many carbs are in everything you put in your mouth!

Ketogenic, Atkins, low-carb paleo, and carnivore diet enthusiasts will have you believing that carbs are the root of all evil, while vegans and pro-metabolic supporters promise that a primarily carbohydrate-rich diet will reward you with the best bill of good health. But the real question is, How many carbs do *you* need to lose weight and feel great? This depends on how much muscle you have (men often can tolerate more carbs than women because they typically have more muscle mass), how much and how hard you work out, your age, and the current state of your metabolic health.

To simplify this process, I only want you to think in terms of *starchy carbs*. This is your bread, rice, pasta, potatoes, tortillas, couscous, quinoa, lentils, and beans. Now, of course you're going to eat small amounts of carbs whenever you eat nonstarchy vegetables, avocados, olives, nuts, seeds, and dairy products, and I do not want you paying attention to any of the carbohydrates found in those foods. We are only looking at the starchy carbs. I also only want you to think in terms of *servings*, not grams:

One serving of starchy carbs = 30–40 grams of carbs.

This range leaves room for other carbohydrate sources in the meal and keeps you below the average carbohydrate threshold. Keeping carbs in this range—along with eating PHFF—will prevent a blood sugar spike and insulin rush. First, let's see what 30–40 grams of starchy carbs looks like.

ONE SERVING OF STARCHY CARBS (30-40 g)

- 3/4 cup cooked rice
- 3/4 cup cooked quinoa
- 1 cup cooked lentils
- 3/4 cup cooked beans
- 2 oz dry chickpea pasta
- 1 large banana
- 2 1/2 cups mixed fruit
- 6 cups air-popped popcorn
- 1/2 cup uncooked steel-cut oats
- 2 slices of bread
- 1 medium potato
- 2 servings of Birch Benders paleo pancake mix

◆   3 Birch Benders frozen waffles

Next, let's determine how many servings of starchy carbs you should shoot for. This chart is a starting point for determining how many servings of starchy carbs your body needs daily. For weight loss, I have found that the majority of my clients do well on two servings of starchy carbs per day, assuming no medical conditions and assuming that they are strength training three or more days per week.

DAILY CARBOHYDRATE GUIDELINES

◆   1 serving of starchy carbs: 30–40 g
◆   Strength training <3 times per week: 1 serving of starchy carbs
◆   Blood-sugar-control issues (PCOS, insulin resistance, type 2 diabetes): 1 serving of starchy carbs
◆   Strength training 3+ times per week: 2 servings of starchy carbs
◆   Athletes, pregnant and breastfeeding women: 3+ servings of starchy carbs

The bottom line with carbs is that the amount of carbs your body needs is highly individualized. It's so important to listen to your body and be constantly checking in. As someone who is strength training three or more times per week and trying to maintain my weight, I often eat three servings of starchy carbs per day because I know that's what it takes to feel my best. Use the chart as a starting point. Your carbohydrate needs can change as you move through weight loss and other life phases, like pregnancy, breastfeeding, aging, stressful times, different workout regimens, hormone imbalances, and medical conditions.

This may sound overwhelming, but as you start to implement what you read in this book, you'll become more and more in tune with your body every single day. For instance, a prime example of needing to eat more carbs is feeling fatigued and struggling to get through workouts. This is a sign that you may need a second starchy carb on your rest days as well. And if you're already doing that, you might need a third starchy carb on the days you work out. Another example is waking up in the middle of the night, especially around 2:00 to 4:00 a.m. (more on this connection in chapter 5).

Any symptoms you are experiencing could, of course, have a totally different root cause (if you're waking up during the night, you might ask yourself, *Am I sleeping enough? Am I eating enough during the day? Is there a hormone issue?*). This is why it's so important to understand how your body works. Once you know how it *should* work, you can start making decisions to support that, instead of writing off the symptoms and thinking that you're "getting old" (everyone's favorite excuse for feeling like shit).

PUTTING IT ALL TOGETHER: THE BYO MEAL GUIDE

This is a grab-and-go BYO Meal Guide: all you have to do is grab from each category and be on your way.

BYO MEAL GUIDE

SMOOTHIE

PROTEIN (1):
- protein powder (30 g protein)
- collagen powder (30 g protein)
- protein powder (20 g) + collagen powder (10 g)
- 1 cup plain Greek yogurt
- 1 cup cottage cheese

HEALTHY FAT (1–3):
- 3 tbsp canned coconut milk, unsweetened
- 2 tbsp coconut flakes, unsweetened
- 2 tbsp heavy cream
- 1/2 cup avocado, sliced
- 2 tsp coconut oil
- 2 tbsp hemp seeds
- 1 tbsp almond butter
- 1 tbsp cashew butter
- 1 tbsp peanut butter
- 3 tbsp pumpkin seeds
- 2 tbsp almonds
- 2 tbsp cashews
- 2 tbsp pecans, halves
- 3 tbsp pistachios, kernels

FIBER (2 OR 3):
- 1 tbsp chia seeds
- 1 tbsp acacia fiber
- 2 tsp inulin fiber
- 1 tbsp flaxseed
- 1 cup frozen cauliflower rice
- 1 cup shredded carrot
- 2 cups spinach
- 2 tbsp cacao powder
- 1/2 cup blackberries
- 1/2 cup raspberries
- 1 cup blueberries
- 1 cup strawberries
- 1/2 cup pumpkin puree

NON-HIGH-FIBER FRUIT (0 OR 1):
- 1/2 banana
- 1/2 cup oranges

- 1/2 cup cherries
- 1/2 cup pineapple
- 1/2 cup peaches
- 1/2 cup pears
- 1/2 cup apples

EXTRAS (UNLIMITED):
- lemon juice
- lime juice
- vanilla extract
- almond extract
- cinnamon
- sea salt
- nutmeg
- mint leaves
- ginger
- turmeric
- Matcha
- dry coffee grounds

BREAKFAST

PROTEIN (1):
- 3 eggs + collagen powder (10 g protein)
- 3 eggs + 3 pieces of bacon
- 2 eggs + 2 oz chicken sausage
- 2 eggs + 2 egg whites + collagen powder (10 g protein)
- 2 eggs + 2 oz steak
- 1 cup plain Greek yogurt + collagen powder (10 g protein)
- 1 cup cottage cheese + collagen powder (10 g protein)
- 6 oz plain Greek yogurt + 1 hard-boiled egg + beef stick

- 5 oz smoked salmon
- 4 oz ground turkey
- 1 cup whole milk + chocolate collagen powder (20 g protein)

HEALTHY FAT (1–3):
- 1/2 cup avocado, sliced
- 2 tsp avocado oil
- 2 tsp olive oil
- 2 tsp coconut oil
- 1 tbsp butter
- 3 tbsp pumpkin seeds
- 3 tbsp almonds, cashews, pecans, walnuts, pistachio kernels, or peanuts
- 1 tbsp almond butter
- 1 tbsp cashew butter
- 1 tbsp peanut butter
- 2 slices bacon
- 1.5 oz pork sausage
- 1/4 cup grain-free granola
- 2 tbsp coconut flakes, unsweetened

FIBER (2 OR 3):
- 1 cup nonstarchy vegetables
- 1 cup strawberries
- 1/2 cup blackberries
- 1/2 cup raspberries
- 1 cup blueberries
- 1 tbsp chia seeds
- 1 tbsp acacia fiber
- 2 tsp inulin fiber
- 1 tbsp flaxseed

STARCHY CARBS—OPTIONAL (30–40 g CARBS; BE SURE TO CHECK LABEL FOR EXACT AMOUNT):

- 2 slices of bread
- 1/2 cup uncooked steel-cut oats
- 2 tortillas
- 3/4 cup diced potatoes
- 1 English muffin
- 1 serving pancakes (e.g., Birch Benders)
- 2–3 waffles (e.g., Birch Benders)

LUNCH

PROTEIN (1):

- 5 oz raw / 3.5 oz cooked chicken breast
- 6 oz nitrate-free deli turkey
- 5 oz can of tuna
- 5.5 oz raw / 4 oz cooked 90%-lean ground beef
- 6 oz raw / 4.5 oz cooked salmon
- 4 oz ground chicken
- 4 oz ground turkey
- 6 oz raw / 4.5 oz cooked shrimp
- 5.5 oz raw / 4 oz cooked chicken thighs
- 1 cup cottage cheese

HEALTHY FAT (1–3):

- 1 oz cheese
- 1/2 cup avocado, sliced
- 1 tbsp mayo
- 2 tsp olive oil
- 2 tsp avocado oil
- 2 tsp coconut oil
- 1 tbsp butter
- 3 tbsp pumpkin seeds

- 20 large olives
- 2 tbsp cream cheese
- 1/4 cup sour cream
- 1/2 cup hummus
- 1 tbsp pesto
- 1/3 cup guacamole

FIBER (UNLIMITED):
- asparagus
- green beans
- beets
- broccoli
- brussels sprouts
- cabbage
- carrots
- cauliflower
- celery
- turnips
- water chestnuts
- zucchini
- squash (any kind)
- cucumber
- eggplant
- collard greens
- kale
- leeks
- mushrooms
- okra
- onion
- peppers
- radishes
- rutabaga
- spinach

STARCHY CARBS—OPTIONAL (30–40 g CARBS):

- 3/4 cup cooked white or brown rice
- 2 servings crackers
- 2 slices of sourdough bread
- 2 oz dry lentil or chickpea pasta
- 3/4 cup baby red potatoes
- 3/4 cup cooked quinoa
- 1 cup cooked lentils
- 3/4 cup cooked chickpeas
- 2 small tortillas
- 1 large (2-inch diameter, 5–7 inches long) sweet potato
- 3/4 cup cooked beans (pinto, kidney, black, northern, etc.)

EXTRAS (UNLIMITED UNLESS OTHERWISE NOTED):

- pickles
- lemon juice
- lime juice
- vinegar (balsamic, apple cider, white, rice, red wine, etc.)
- miso
- sauerkraut
- Dijon mustard
- mustard
- barbecue sauce (1–2 tbsp)
- ketchup (1–2 tbsp)
- herbs
- seasonings
- coconut aminos
- soy sauce

DINNER

PROTEIN (1):
- 5.5 oz raw / 4 oz cooked 90%-lean ground beef
- 6 oz raw / 4.5 oz cooked salmon
- 4 oz cooked cod, halibut, or tilapia
- 4 oz ground chicken
- 5 oz raw / 3.5 oz cooked chicken breast
- 6 medium oysters
- 5.5 oz raw / 4 oz cooked pork chop or tenderloin
- 5.5 oz raw / 4 oz cooked 90%-lean ground turkey
- 6 oz raw / 4.5 oz cooked shrimp
- 8.5 oz raw / 5 oz cooked scallops
- 6 oz raw / 4 oz cooked sirloin

HEALTHY FAT (1–3):
- 1 oz cheese
- 1/2 cup avocado, sliced
- 1 tbsp mayo
- 2 tsp olive oil
- 2 tsp avocado oil
- 2 tsp coconut oil
- 1 tbsp butter
- 3 tbsp pumpkin seeds
- 20 large olives
- 2 tbsp cream cheese
- 1/4 cup sour cream
- 1/2 cup hummus
- 1 tbsp pesto
- 1/3 cup guacamole

FIBER (UNLIMITED):
- artichoke
- asparagus

- green beans
- beets
- broccoli
- brussels sprouts
- cabbage
- carrots
- cauliflower
- celery
- turnips
- water chestnuts
- zucchini
- squash (any kind)
- cucumber
- eggplant
- collard greens
- kale
- leeks
- mushrooms
- okra
- onion
- peppers
- radishes
- rutabaga
- spinach
- sauerkraut

STARCHY CARBS—OPTIONAL (30–40 g CARBS):
- 1 cup cooked corn
- 1 1/4 cup cooked peas
- 3/4 cup cooked white or brown rice
- 2 oz dry lentil or chickpea pasta
- 3/4 cup baby red potatoes
- 3/4 cup cooked quinoa
- 1 cup cooked lentils
- 1 cup refried beans

- 3/4 cup cooked barley
- 1 cup cooked couscous
- 1 cup cooked wild rice
- 2 slices of bread
- 2 small tortillas
- 1 large (2-inch diameter, 5–7 inches long) sweet potato
- 3/4 cup cooked beans (pinto, kidney, black, northern, etc.)

SNACKS (15–30 g PROTEIN, 10–20 g FAT, 0–30 g CARBS):

Snacks are variable based on your hunger and how long they will need to sustain you until your next meal.

PROTEIN (1 OR 2):
- 1/2 cup cottage cheese
- 3/4 cup plain Greek yogurt
- protein powder (20–25 g protein)
- 2 beef sticks
- 2 hard-boiled eggs
- 1 cup edamame, shelled
- 2 pieces of string cheese
- 2 oz prosciutto
- 3 oz nitrate-free deli turkey
- 3 oz can of tuna
- 2 oz chopped cooked chicken breast

HEALTHY FAT (1 OR 2):
- 1/3 cup guacamole
- 3 tbsp pumpkin seeds
- 1/2 cup avocado, sliced
- 2 tbsp cream cheese
- 1 oz cheese
- 20 large olives

- 2 tbsp coconut flakes, unsweetened
- 1/4 cup grain-free granola
- 1/2 cup hummus
- 2 oz salami
- 1 tbsp mayo
- 2 tbsp almonds
- 2 tbsp cashews
- 2 tbsp pecans, halves
- 3 tbsp pistachios, kernels
- 1 tbsp almond butter
- 1 tbsp cashew butter
- 1 tbsp peanut butter

OPTIONAL ADD-ONS (1):
- nonstarchy vegetables
- 1 serving crackers
- 1/2 cup berries
- 2–3 rice cakes
- 1 serving tortilla chips
- 1 tbsp chia seeds
- 1 tbsp acacia fiber
- 2 tsp inulin fiber
- 2 tbsp flaxseed
- 2 tbsp cacao powder
- 1/2 cup berries
- 1/2 banana
- 1/2 cup frozen fruit
- 1/2 cup pumpkin puree

ON-THE-GO BARS:
- RXBAR
- Nash Bar
- No Cow
- Bhu Foods
- Paleovalley
- Kion Bar

PAST DIETER PROFILE

Carol was a highly seasoned dieter—Atkins, the grapefruit diet, Jenny Craig, WeightWatchers—and survived off cigarettes and TaB. She started her first diet when she was just 12 years old. When Carol was in her sixties, she started eating PHFF and lost 11 inches eating more food than she ever had before. Not only that but her entire mindset and attitude around food changed. She feels more confident and happy in every aspect of her life and has no plans to ever go on another diet again.

How to Adjust the BYO Meal Guide

I know there are a lot of numbers in this chapter, and that can be intimidating. But, remember, those numbers are not meant to limit you; they are meant to empower you. I want you to know exactly what to eat for your optimal metabolic health. There is no need to be militant—your body is not a math equation, after all. But if you just gained awareness that you're severely undereating protein and over-eating carbohydrates, you can make that change starting tomorrow. Armed with this info, you can make it easily!

While there may be a bit of a learning curve as you begin to read labels and check the charts for serving sizes, this will eventually become so second nature that you won't need to measure a thing. Use the following framework to help determine how much food your body needs to restore optimal function and begin to lose fat:

1. Calculate your daily protein requirement, decide how many meals you'll eat each day, and determine your protein goal for each meal. (To recap, the simple starting point to help calculate your protein requirement is 0.8 x body weight or 1 x weight at a BMI of 25.)
2. Find your carbohydrate starting point (one, two, or three or more servings of starchy carbs per day).

3. Use the BYO Meal Guide to build your meals with protein, healthy fat, fiber, and carbs.
   - Include a protein that meets your protein goals.
   - Include one to three servings of healthy fat. Stick to one to two servings if you're having a starchy carb, and two to three servings if you're not having a starchy carb.
   - Include fiber at each meal. Don't obsess over numbers, but if your goal is 25 grams of fiber per day, you'll want to shoot for about 8 grams of fiber per meal.
   - Include one serving of a starchy carb (optional, depending on carb requirements).
4. If a meal doesn't keep you satisfied for four hours, it's time to add more food!
   - Are you eating your recommended protein amount?
   - Are you eating enough fiber?
   - If yes to the above, it's time to add another serving of fat!
5. Do you feel satiated but are getting tired and sluggish, especially during workouts? Are you finding that your performance is slipping during workouts? It's likely time to add another starchy carb!

Let's see what this might look like in practice. If your 8:00 a.m. smoothie has 30 grams of protein, chia seeds, and raspberries for fiber and one serving of almond butter for fat but you're hungry by 10:00 a.m., try adding a second serving of almond butter tomorrow and see how that makes you feel. Once you can make it until lunch without needing to eat, you've hit the jackpot. You're eating the amount of food your body needs to fuel itself properly.

One final important point to make before we close this chapter: in the beginning, your hunger and satiety signals may be out of sync. So, even though I'm teaching you how to trust your body and read its signals, you may not be in a place right now where you're able to do that. That's okay, and I have some tips to help you get started.

If you're someone who never feels hungry, it's likely because your body has slowed down to preserve energy from an extended period of calorie deprivation. But the good news is that your body is in a constant state of flux. Your metabolism will rev back up, and your hunger signals will return as you begin to feed your body regularly again. Start with breakfast (as in, eat breakfast!), even if it's something small.

If you're someone who always feels hungry, never fear—as you begin to balance your blood sugar, you will quickly start to feel more satiated throughout the day. Eat PHFF at every meal for three days, and if you still feel hungry all the time, you'll know that you're just not eating enough and it's time to refer to the "How to Adjust the BYO Meal Guide" section and increase your food intake.

Whoa, that was a lot of new, exciting information. Starting on any new journey comes with a certain amount of fear or anxiety. I get that! That's why I offer these guidelines and give you the tools to adjust them depending on where you are right now. Think of this chapter as your walking stick: it will give you that extra bit of stability and support to trek ahead without any fear of falling.

30-SECOND SUMMARY

If you're feeling overwhelmed, don't! Read this chapter again. Perhaps try it in small sections, or read it out loud. And while you're reading, practice by focusing on the following to keep blood sugar steady, your body burning fat, and your belly satiated all day long:

1. **Eat PHFF:** First and foremost, start incorporating PHFF into each meal. This will maintain nice and steady blood sugar levels, burn fat, and keep your metabolism lit.

2. **Eat when you're hungry:** You know you better than I do—or any other diet "guru" for that matter. Don't skip meals, and don't eat so little that you're hungry in a couple of hours. Your meals should be keeping you satisfied for a full four hours. If they're not, you need to eat more! Start to really listen to your body and recognize when it's hungry and when it's not, and you'll start to see amazing results.

3. **Don't eat carbs naked:** Even if you can't make your meal PHFF for whatever reason, do your best to not eat carbs

alone. Always eat some peanut butter with that banana or cheese with those crackers; it'll still slow down the uptake of sugar into your system.

Shifting your mindset from counting calories, tracking macros, and eliminating food groups to managing your BS is the first step toward taking back your power over food. In the next chapter, I'm going to shift your mindset yet again, from a focus on fat loss to muscle gain, and this new shift is going to change the way you approach your body forever.

CHAPTER 3

MUSCLE IS MONEY

Have you ever been on a diet where you're told that as you lose weight, you'll have to adjust your calorie intake downward to maintain that weight loss? Or have you ever been told that when you hit a plateau, it means it's time to drop your calories even further?

There are two reasons for this:

1. Metabolic adaptation: Your body adjusts to the lower calorie intake and, consequently, lowers the number of calories it's burning each day (this is the body's neat survival technique experienced by Alex in chapter 1).
2. Loss of lean muscle: Low-calorie diets result in a loss of lean muscle, and as you lose muscle, your metabolic rate drops. You eat less and less to maintain your weight loss, making it more and more difficult to maintain it.

No wonder most people who go on a reduced-calorie diet end up gaining the weight back (and then some) in the end. To add insult to injury, most old-school diets push cardio for a high-calorie burn. These long, high-intensity cardio sessions—especially when done regularly—are a form of stress on the body that sends the signal that you're seeking endurance instead of strength. In return, your body will adapt and become efficient for endurance exercise in two ways:

1. You'll begin to shed unnecessary weight *from your muscles*. Excess muscle isn't needed for endurance exercise, so it's deadweight to a body being primed for long bouts of cardio. And because muscle is denser than fat, it makes sense for your body to prioritize shedding it.
2. You'll begin to store easily accessible energy *in your fat cells*. Fat is a good storage facility for the energy needed for long-form cardio, and it has unlimited storage space.

Long, high-intensity workouts like boot camps, spin classes, and six-mile runs may burn a lot of calories on your Apple Watch, but doing these types of workouts every day—especially when you're in a calorie deficit—will eventually make the body more efficient at burning those calories. This means that although your watch may say you burned 600 calories in a workout, your body actually may have only burned 100 calories.

PAST DIETER PROFILE

Erin had been a client of mine for several months. She was eating PHFF, sleeping well, doing her best to manage stress with two kids and a full-time job, and running four days per week, but she wasn't seeing any changes in her body. I told Erin it was time to back off the running and incorporate more strength training. In one week, she swapped her runs for weights and dropped three pounds. It wasn't three pounds of fat, but some of that weight came from the water her body was holding on to due to the high levels of cortisol being triggered by overexercising. You'll learn more about cortisol, and the damage it can do to our metabolic health when chronically raised, in chapter 6.

There are a lot of wonderful benefits to cardiovascular exercise, but long-term fat loss is not one of them. If you enjoy cardio as a part of your fitness routine, great—don't stop. But be honest with yourself. If you're sweating it out for fat loss, your long-term ROI will be disappointing.

Dr. Gabrielle Lyon of Muscle-Centric Medicine says that "we are not overfat, we are undermuscled" (Power and Rupsis 2021 [see "Macronutrients" in references]). This is such an empowering point of view because it gives you total voluntary control over moving and growing your muscles.

To get the most reward with the least amount of effort, it's time to stop focusing on burning as many calories as possible during your workouts and to start focusing on burning as many calories as possible *all day long* by increasing your muscle mass.

Let's dive into why having more muscle is the key to biologically setting you up for long-term weight loss and how to build muscle by spending far less time in the gym than you'd ever imagine.

WHY YOU NEED MORE MUSCLE

The reasons to build muscle are endless, but for the purposes of this book, we'll be focusing on the fact that the more muscle you have on your body, the more calories you'll burn lying around watching Netflix—no joke!

Your skeletal muscle mass composes 30–40 percent of your total body weight. These are the muscles that connect to your bones and allow you to perform daily movements and functions. They also look nice in tank tops, have anti-inflammatory properties, and are our largest site for glucose disposal (i.e., they soak up the carbohydrates we eat).

Let's first take a look at how your body burns calories daily.

Your total daily energy expenditure (TDEE) is the number of calories your body requires to maintain weight and keep you alive and well. This chart breaks down how those calories are being used.

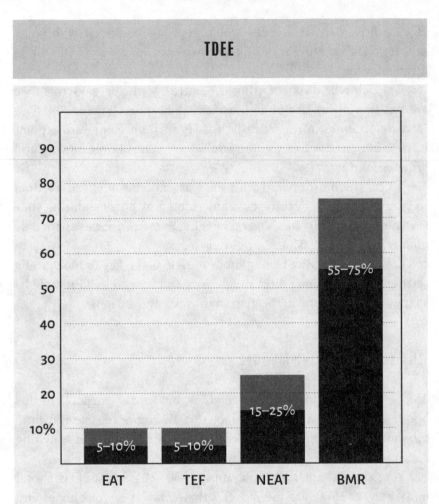

We often think about our total expenditure as the amount of energy we burn at the gym and through our daily activities, but you can see by looking at this chart that exercise activity thermogenesis (EAT)—that is, the calories burned during exercise—only makes up around 5–10 percent of our daily burn.

Your basal metabolic rate (BMR), on the other hand, makes up 55–75 percent of your daily calorie burn. These are the calories you would need to consume even if you were in a coma, just to keep your organs going. It does not include any of the basic activities you perform throughout the day! So, if you're beating yourself up about skipping the gym, know that you're still burning a hell of a lot of calories every day.

Next, we have nonexercise activity thermogenesis (NEAT), which is all the walking, fidgeting, cleaning, standing versus sitting, and other movement you do every day to get things done. These are the calories you're burning by living your life. It does not include hitting the weights at the gym or spinning like crazy on a stationary bike (that's EAT). Notice that this is a bigger chunk of your calorie burn than your designated workout time.

Next up is TEF. We touched on this in the last chapter when we discussed the high TEF of protein. TEF is the number of calories burned each day just through the digestion of food. Yes, digestion is *that* taxing! Protein has the highest TEF because it takes the longest to break down and digest.

The most important takeaway from this chart, however, is that while exercise is important, increasing your BMR will give you the biggest bang for your metabolic buck. This is where your muscles become the star of the show. Muscle is calorically expensive to maintain, so the body has to burn a lot of calories just to keep it. More muscle means a higher BMR, which means more calories burned at rest. That's right: just having more muscle means you burn more calories by doing nothing at all.

BUILD AND MAINTAIN MUSCLE

Muscle is metabolic money. The more muscle we have, the more calories we burn at rest, the more food we can eat, and the more "metabolically flexible" we are. We'll talk about metabolic flexibility in the next chapter, but what's important to know here is that the more metabolically flexible you are, the more you're able to be flexible with your food choices and exercise routine without weight gain.

We build and maintain muscle in two ways:

1. Through activation of *muscle protein synthesis* by consuming enough amino acids via the protein in our diet
2. Through *strength training*—also known as muscle activation

Muscle Protein Synthesis

Amino acids are the building blocks for protein. There are 20 types of amino acids, but only nine of them are "essential," meaning we must consume them through food in order to both survive *and* thrive.

Muscle protein synthesis—or muscle building—occurs only when our bodies have consumed enough essential amino acids. There is one primary amino acid, called leucine, that jump-starts the muscle protein synthesis process, but we truly need all nine to complete it. Animal proteins, like steak, chicken, and eggs, contain large amounts of essential amino acids to easily trigger muscle protein synthesis. As a rule of thumb, as long as you are consuming 30 grams of animal protein in a meal, you are probably triggering muscle growth and repair. Plant-based proteins, like soy, lentils, and beans, have far fewer essential amino acids, making them less optimal for muscle growth.

Now, this doesn't mean that eating less than 30 grams in a meal or eating plant-based protein is a waste. Protein is responsible for nearly all the work that is carried out in every cell, so consuming adequate protein daily—whether it's through eggs, meat, lentils, tofu, or any other protein-rich food—will do a body *very* good. But getting that 30 grams of animal protein will trigger muscle growth all day long, not just during your workouts.

A good trick if you consume no or a limited amount of animal products is to find a plant-based protein powder with added leucine or added essential amino acids and make a shake for breakfast. These are often classified as "sports" protein powders that are designed with your muscles in mind.

Strength Training

The simplest, surefire way to build muscle is to strength train, which just means moving your muscles through heavy resistance.

Before we get into why it works (and what it is), it's important to understand that strength training comes with a mindset adjustment. Especially when it comes to women and weight loss, strength training is one of the most underrated and misunderstood tools. When most women think about weight lifting, they think about bodybuilders, steroids, grunting, and tan, oiled physiques. Let's all move past that image, shall we? We can paint a more accurate picture.

The point of *strength* training is to get stronger. And while that seems obvious, it is a bit counterintuitive as a strategy when your goal is burning as many calories as possible so you can lose weight. Set that aside. Your new goal is gaining strength—something that goes beyond weight loss and can help you in every aspect of your life. And speaking of going beyond weight loss, you don't have to ditch cardio altogether to see results. The point of this chapter is to help you understand how vitally important building strength is not only for your metabolism but also for your overall health and longevity. We'll dig more into how specific types of cardiovascular exercise affect your metabolism in the next chapter.

PAST DIETER PROFILE

Rochelle was a brand-new client and, at 65 years old, had never lifted a weight in her life, despite having a very active lifestyle. After completing a 12-week strength-training program, she had gone up in weight in every exercise, felt stronger, and was seeing sexy muscle definition for the first time in her life.

You've probably used the scale as your primary measurement of progress in the past, but the scale provides very little information about a far more relevant parameter of health (and what you look like naked), which is your body composition.

Often, clients who begin strength training only wanting to lose 5–10 pounds see very little to no movement on the scale. This is because they are steadily gaining muscle as they drop fat, and the scale does not discriminate between muscle mass and fat mass. Thus, taking measurements or tracking pictures of yourself, instead of daily weigh-ins, is so important to assessing progress.

Here are some dos and don'ts for taking measurements and tracking with pictures:

1. Don't do it daily. Just as your body weight on the scale can fluctuate up to 1–2 percent every day, your measurements, especially around your midsection, can change, too, based on what you've eaten, how hydrated you are, how intense your exercise was, and your monthly cycle (if you have one).

2. Do wear the same clothes and use the same lighting in the same mirror for taking photos. Even subtle variations in clothing style and color can make a difference. This goes for taking measurements, too, if you're measuring with clothes on.

3. Don't only measure around the waist. We all lose, and hold on to, fat in different areas of our bodies based on genetics. If you tend to carry more weight in your midsection, you will get discouraged if progress is slower there. I recommend choosing three to five spots to measure consistently, like the waist, hips, thighs, chest, and upper arms.

4. Do give yourself time to see progress by only measuring or taking photos once per month. This can be difficult if you're used to weighing every day, but if you're someone who gets easily discouraged by not seeing overnight results, this is a way to really create positive habits without the stress of tracking progress.

TRACKING BODY COMPOSITION AT HOME:

HOW TO TAKE PROGRESS MEASUREMENTS

1. **Waist:** Line up the tape measure with your belly button, and make sure it's level all the way around your body. Make sure you are not taking this measurement around the time of your period because it will likely be inaccurate.

2. **Hips:** It's a little easier to think of this as measuring around your butt. Find the widest part of your hips, which will likely be right across your bum, and measure.

3. **Thigh:** As done with your hips, you'll measure around the widest part of your leg, which will be toward the very top of your leg.

4. **Chest:** Line up the tape measure with your nipples, and take the measurement underneath your arms. This one is a little more difficult if you have breasts, because you want to be sure you're not smashing them down. Just fit the measuring tape comfortably around your bust.

5. **Upper arm:** From the tip of the elbow, measure six inches up the arm, and take your measurement around the arm there.

While adding strength training may not result in a dramatic drop in weight right away, you will look different. And so far in my career, I haven't heard a single complaint about this.

Strength training can include using free weights, barbells, weight machines, resistance bands, or even one's own body weight. What's important is allowing your muscles to spend time under tension and working toward getting stronger.

So, no matter what techniques or kinds of weights you use, you are performing progressive overload, meaning you are increasing your weight or reps every week. If you're using your body weight, you're not doing 20 push-ups every other day—you're doing 20, then 21, then 22.

In order to continue building muscle, you must continue to challenge those muscles. If you don't progressively overload your training, you'll struggle to build lean muscle.

Remember, your focus is no longer a calorie burn—your focus is getting stronger. As long as that remains in the front of your mind, you *will see* results.

CREATE A WORKOUT ROUTINE

When it comes to exercise, there are generally two groups of people: those who make working out a top priority and wouldn't dream of skipping a workout, regardless of their busy schedule, and those who consistently leave exercise off the table because they simply don't have the time and can't prioritize it.

If you're in the second camp, it's usually because you figure, What's the point of starting an exercise routine if you can't make it to the gym five or six days a week? But it takes a lot less time than you think to establish a consistent routine that will help you build strength. Let's take a look.

1. If you've never done strength training before or if you're in the "I simply do not have time" camp:
    • Start by doing two or three 30–60-minute full-body workouts each week. You do not need to do more to see results. I hit the gym on Saturday and Sunday to take advantage of day care and then one more time during the week on my least busy day.
    • Track your weights and/or reps so that you can slowly increase in weight and/or reps each week—a little more weight or one more rep. The notes app on your phone works great.
    • *Take rest days.* Two minimum.
    • Make sure you're consuming enough protein to support these new muscle fibers. Follow the protein guidelines in chapter 2.

2. If you're not new to strength training and you're ready to take it to the next level:
   - Plan to train three or four days per week. If you do three days, do full-body workouts. If you do four days, split your training between upper-body days and lower-body days.
   - Follow the remaining guidelines from number one above.
   - Other progressive overload programs that I love are from Mind Pump Media, Paragon Training Methods, Moves by Madeline, and Sohee Fit.

Need more structure? Great! Here is an example of a one-month full-body training program to get you started. Repeat this full workout three days a week for four weeks in a row, increasing in reps or weight each week. You can keep track of reps and weight in a notes app to make sure you're increasing your load each week. This workout can be done at home or at a gym with a few sets of dumbbells or resistance bands. If you aren't sure how to do some of these exercises, head to the Metabolism Makeover website (metabolismmakeover.co/resources) for videos of each one.

DAY 1

- split squats: 2 sets of 8–12 reps
- bent-over rows: 3 sets of 8–12 reps
- bench press: 3 sets of 8–12 reps
- Romanian dead lift: 4 sets of 8–12 reps
- push-ups: 3 sets of 10–15 reps
- bicep curls: 3 sets of 10–15 reps

DAY 2

- bench step-ups: 2 sets of 12–15 reps
- glute bridge: 2 sets of 12–15 reps
- sissy squats: 2 sets of 8–15 reps
- leaning lateral raise: 3 sets of 10–15 reps
- banded lateral raise: 3 sets of 10–15 reps
- overhead tricep extension: 2 sets of 10–15 reps

DAY 3

- front squats: 2 sets of 12–15 reps
- overhead press: 3 sets of 8–12 reps
- chest flies: 2 sets of 12–15 reps
- one-arm bent-over rows: 2 sets of 10–12 reps per arm
- upright rows: 2 sets of 10–15 reps
- V-ups: 1 minute
- reverse crunches: 1 minute

STRENGTH-TRAINING FAQS

1. Won't I get bulky?

It's highly unlikely that you will look bulky from strength training alone unless you're taking hormones to put on size. "Getting big" is typically connected to a hell of a lot of testosterone that women simply do not have. Genetics can play a role here, too, but muscle growth happens *very* slowly, especially in women.

2. What if I really can't work out?

Whether you have an injury or a health condition or you're in a season of life that simply doesn't allow you to exercise, remember the 80/20 rule. Hone in on the other pillars, especially your diet, and pay close attention to blood sugar balance. Adjust carbohydrate intake as needed, based on what you learned in chapter 2. And, remember, to trigger muscle protein synthesis, you'll need to consume at least 30 grams of animal protein (or a plant-based protein powder with added amino acids) per meal. Protein will be vitally important to maintaining the muscle mass you already have.

3. Does my favorite barre class count?

Exercise is better than no exercise. Movement is better than no movement. Moving your body and your muscles on a regular basis is key to feeling good and confident in your body.

But if your goal is to increase your BMR and burn fat by adding muscle to your body, workouts that focus on accessory muscles, flexibility, and stability—like barre, yoga, and Pilates—will not give you the biggest bang for your metabolic buck. These can be fabulous complements to your resistance-training routine, as they do offer great benefits. But the goal with these workouts should not be fat loss.

30-SECOND SUMMARY

Muscle is metabolic money in that the more muscle we have, the more calories we burn at rest and the more food we can eat without weight gain!

1. **Resistance train:** First and foremost, get your muscles under tension. This could be lifting weights, using resistance bands, or even just using your own body weight.
2. **Take rest days:** A great way to never see progress at the gym is spending every day at the gym. Take a minimum of two days per week to rest.

3. **Eat protein at every meal:** Getting at least 30 grams of animal protein in a meal triggers muscle protein synthesis. Do this three times a day and you'll be in good shape for triggering muscle growth. If you're avoiding animal products, use a plant-based protein powder with added essential amino acids once per day.

Now that you understand how different types of workouts affect whether you'll burn calories *all day* (through building lean muscle) or *only in your workout sessions* (through lots of cardio), let's step it up a notch. In the next chapter, you'll learn how different types of movement—outside of the gym—affect your metabolic health, blood sugar response, stress levels, and even how you age.

CHAPTER 4

LIVING IN MOTION

I would venture to guess that the majority of you reading this book would not consider yourselves to be sedentary, especially if you're a regular gym goer.

If you hit the gym five or six times per week for an hour but then get your groceries and dinner delivered while sitting at your desk or lie on the couch or bed for the remaining 23 hours, you fall into the category of *actively* sedentary. Which is really just a way of saying, *You're sedentary—but here's a gold star for your workout today.*

Why does this matter? Well, you know all those studies that tell us a sedentary lifestyle has a negative impact on nearly every aspect of human health? That sitting at a desk all day automatically increases your risk of obesity, chronic disease, and early death? That's you—you're in that category, even if you're exercising regularly. I know this is harsh news, but I'm here to help get you on a better path.

The adverse health effects of a sedentary lifestyle are rooted in two factors:

1. Burning fewer calories from our natural movements
2. Keeping the body in one position for a prolonged period of time

Burning fewer calories really isn't a problem as long as we're not overconsuming. But if you're actively trying to lose weight, this can make things especially difficult, since NEAT movement makes up 15–25 percent of our daily calorie burn (see chapter 3). The main problem, though, isn't that we're just not getting enough steps in every day. It's that we're just *not moving*. We're glued to our desk/computer/TV, and it's making us sick, overweight, and immobile later in life.

In this chapter, I'll walk through why movement is key to a healthy body and weight as you age, how much you really need, and the simple ways to increase movement enough in your day to go from actively sedentary to active, even if you're tied to a desk.

WHAT COUNTS AS MOVEMENT?

Everyone has a different definition of movement, but I define it as *living in motion*. It's any low-impact physical activity—mostly nonexercise movement like walking, housework, gardening, hiking, squatting down to pick up your toddler or a heavy box, standing at your desk instead of sitting, or even fidgeting—but it can also include moving from one position to another to avoid remaining in the same position all day. We don't consider these to be exercise, but they move our bodies daily.

Aside from a sedentary lifestyle contributing to early death, movement is important for metabolic flexibility, blood sugar control, stress relief, and—my personal favorite—the ability to *maintain movement as we age*.

Metabolic Flexibility

Workouts go through trends just like anything else. And some are better than others. In the '90s, we were told to "stay in the fat-burning zone" with our cardio workouts. Stop sprinting on the treadmill, start incline walking! In the 2000s, we moved toward high-intensity interval training and an obsession with workout calorie burn. But it turns out that we were onto something with "fat-burning zone" cardio.

Let's go back to biology class for a minute. Remember all that energy we're creating by eating PHFF? Well, our mitochondria are the specific part of our cells that generate that energy. When we have healthy, abundant mitochondria, our body becomes metabolically flexible, meaning the body's metabolism is adaptable enough to use whatever fuel is available to it. The body can then easily burn fat for energy, instead of always relying on carbohydrates. Those with a sedentary lifestyle tend to be less metabolically flexible, meaning their bodies are more likely to struggle with using fat for energy and often go straight to burning carbohydrates—or glucose—as a fuel source. This is a problem because the body will have a hard time burning fat and will keep its food-seeking mechanisms constantly on because it wants those carbohydrates to use as energy. The good news is that when functioning properly, our mitochondria are easily able to switch from using carbohydrates to using fat as fuel.

So we want to be metabolically flexible, right? While all forms of physical activity are beneficial for overall health, a combination of aerobic cardio and strength training is the key to increasing the healthy mitochondria responsible for increasing the body's metabolic flexibility. We've already discussed strength training, so let's get into cardio. Short for *cardiovascular exercise*, the term *cardio* refers to any exercise that gets your heart pumping for a prolonged period of time. Running, cycling, and stair climbing are common cardio exercises. There are five different zones of heart training, so let's start by defining each:

- Zone 1: 50–60 percent of maximum heart rate—you should be able to easily maintain a conversation here.
- Zone 2: 60–70 percent of maximum heart rate—you should be able to maintain a conversation here, but you're having to pause occasionally to take a breath.
- Zone 3: 70–80 percent of maximum heart rate—you can talk, but you're probably keeping it to one- or two-word answers.
- Zone 4: 80–90 percent of maximum heart rate—you're only able to spurt out one-word answers, and you're not really happy about being asked questions.
- Zone 5: 90–100 percent of maximum heart rate—don't talk to me!

While there are benefits to each zone, zone 2 is where it's at if you want to use fat more efficiently as a fuel source. It's also the zone that brings the body into a more parasympathetic, or relaxed, state. All exercise causes our bodies to release endorphins, or "feel-good" hormones, but low-intensity exercise doesn't increase your heart rate enough to activate the sympathetic (or, fight or flight) nervous system. We often associate practices like meditation or yoga with calming the nervous system, but if that doesn't appeal to you, try walking, light jogging, swimming, bike riding, or dancing instead. The literature tells us that an optimal amount of zone 2 cardio is 150–180 minutes per week, and this could be anywhere from two 90-minute walks to daily 20-minute dance breaks.

Blood Sugar Control: The Movement Edition

The second most effective way to control your blood sugar, after eating PHFF, is moving your body after meals.

Blood sugar levels hit a peak within 90 minutes of eating a meal, and what I know both from research and from using my body as a science experiment via a blood sugar monitor is that a 20-minute walk, jog, or bike ride after a meal can reduce blood sugar spikes. Steady blood sugar equals less insulin equals more fat burn! And, really, any type of exercise can work here. But a walk can be a good multitasker while you're hanging out with your partner or kids after dinner or while on a post-lunch work call.

Stress Relief

While we're on the subject of multitasking, research has shown that taking a stroll—even for just 10 minutes—releases endorphins that stimulate relaxation and an improved mood. And I'm not necessarily talking about zone 2 cardio; even a casual walk around the block after dinner can promote a chill state. And as you'll discover in chapter 6, stress is the number one contributor to weight-loss resistance.

While managing the stress in your mind might be challenging, taking a relaxing walk is a fairly low-barrier activity that most can implement in their daily routine. Bonus if you add sunshine for a dose of serotonin to lift your energy and mood. Bigger bonus if you are on unfamiliar terrain or if you walk barefoot (more on that later in this chapter).

PAST DIETER PROFILE

Jacqueline was so discouraged when she came to me because she had been an avid exerciser her whole life but, due to a medical diagnosis, was unable to exert any effort in her physical activity. She was six months postpartum and was depressed that she wouldn't be able to drop any of the baby weight without the gym. I asked her to very slowly add zone 2 cardio to her daily routine and see how her body responded. It was low impact enough that she got up to two 20-minute walks each day, and within three months, Jacqueline had dropped a pants size and was feeling back to her old self—without the gym.

Get Moving with Intention

At this point, I know you're asking, *So how much movement do I need?* A meta-analysis of 15 international cohorts looked at number of steps per day and mortality; the bottom line was simply that taking more steps was associated with a lower risk of death, up to a level that varied by age.

I hate to be vague, but, as a general rule, the more movement the better. Instead of focusing on hitting a certain number of steps, I want you to constantly be thinking about how you can move more and how you can move *better*:

- If you currently track your steps and are getting in 3,000 steps per day, what would it take to hit 4,000 steps?

- If you don't track, but you know you don't intentionally fit movement into your day, what can you add to your day to do so?

It can be challenging to think of ways to get in more movement if your job requires you to be tied to your desk all day. So I went straight to my community and asked them how they incorporate creative movement into their busy days. Here's what they said! Notice that many of these movement tips are habit stacked with other things you probably already do daily.

1. **Schedule daily walks:** Put a walk into your calendar as a meeting with your body. Twenty to 30 minutes of zone 2 cardio per day is ideal. Or if it works better for your schedule, alternate days at the gym with a 45-minute walk. You can even break these up into several 5–10-minute walks throughout the day. The barrier to entry for walking is so low that many of the suggestions on this list incorporate this form of movement.

2. **Sneak in random movement:** Do push-ups while waiting for the water to heat up in the shower or calf raises while you're brushing your teeth. Hold yoga poses while watching TV. Every hour, get up and go to the bathroom, take a walk around the block or the office, switch out the laundry, or simply get up and wiggle it out for a few. Habit stacking is a fun way to incorporate more movement throughout the day.

3. **Stand 50 percent of the day instead of sitting:** Standing burns 50 percent more calories and reduces post-meal blood sugar levels considerably, compared with sitting. In one study of office workers, standing for 180 minutes after lunch reduced the post-lunch blood sugar spike by 43 percent, compared with sitting for the same amount of time. Another office-worker study discovered that alternating between standing and sitting every 30 minutes throughout the workday reduced blood sugar spikes by 11.1 percent on average.

4. **Involve the kids and pets:** A family walk or bike ride is a fun and connecting after-dinner activity. Dance parties, swimming pool races, and rolling around on the ground with your kids or pets are a few great ways to get the whole family involved.

5. **Get an accountability partner:** We are far more likely to achieve a goal we've set for ourselves with the combination of accountability and a set time to follow through. So grab a friend and hold each other accountable for going on walks, and set a time that works for both of you—even if you can only meet virtually. Bonus: connection is key for well-being and stress management, so you're already getting a jump on chapter 6!

6. **Move more—and differently—at work:** If it's possible, make a commitment to walk or bike to work two or three times a week. Take walking meetings or stand during Zoom calls. Walk to your coworker's desk to ask a question instead of sending an email. Lower your work space and sit on a yoga pillow or in a squat for part of the day or raise it with a standing desk. And if you're working from home, get up and move, put the dishes away, or drop for some floor stretches when you have a few minutes between tasks.

7. **Sit differently:** Our bodies are not meant to be seated in a chair all day long. While this can be impossible to avoid all the time, you can mix up your seating arrangements throughout the day for more movement. Sit on the floor instead of the couch, sit on a yoga pillow, squat, sit cross-legged, sit with your legs stretched out, sit on an exercise ball—sitting options are endless.

8. **Walk differently:** If you truly don't have time to do a 20–30-minute walk every day, squeeze one in when you can and boost the benefits by walking on grass, gravel, or a hill, or even going barefoot. Each experience gives your body a different range of motion to work through with different muscles. A variety of movement is better movement.

9. **Boost natural movement with chores:** Everybody has to do chores, so make them work for you. Use a watering can to water flowers instead of a hose, use a push mower instead of an automatic, and pull out the ole vacuum instead of using a Roomba. Set a timer and turbo clean a space for 10 minutes. Or my personal favorite is rage cleaning. If you don't know what rage cleaning is, you may not be the type of person who aggressively cleans when they need to let off some steam!

10. **Habit stack with other pillars of the Metabolic Ecosystem:** Instead of viewing movement as another thing on your to-do list, view it as something fun that you do every day just for you, as a stress reliever. When you go out for your walk, throw on a podcast, call or meet up with a friend, or zone out to your favorite playlist. One of my favorite habit stacks is taking a walk to get in morning sunlight for better sleep (more on this in chapter 5). You can also make it a habit to go on a 10–20-minute post-meal walk to stabilize blood sugar levels, and as mentioned above, this is a great way to get the family or pets involved. And, finally, keep in mind that more movement means better digestion. Imagine how your poor digestive system feels stuck in that same sitting position all day. Give it a little breathing room!

Katy Bowman, founder of Nutritious Movement, says that a restrictive movement diet is similar to a restrictive food diet. When we eat certain foods, the nutrients in those foods communicate with our bodies and are used in a certain way. Bowman says that movement is similar. The body is affected by the movement that you do (or don't) feed it.

All this means is that I don't just want you to increase your daily steps, although that is an excellent start if you're currently sitting most of the day. What you should be looking to increase is total movement for complete metabolic health and longevity. This might include standing instead of sitting, squatting to pick something up, sitting on the floor to fold laundry, or doing the monkey bars at the park.

Instead of worrying about weight gain as you age, worry about what would *cause* that weight gain. A lowered metabolic rate due to muscle loss and the inability to move and exercise the way you want should be a concern, not arbitrary weight gain.

When thinking about movement as we age, I often think about Dr. Peter Attia's concept of the "marginal decade," that is, the last decade of your life. What do you want your life to look like in your last decade? What do you want to be doing? How do you want to move? You can do something about keeping your body mobile and your muscles intact: you have that power—use it.

Movement's price of admission is *low.* When you compare it with balancing your diet, driving to the gym, picking up a set of dumbbells, disciplining yourself to stop scrolling and get to bed sooner, reducing your stress, or addressing your gut health, moving your body a little more is really simple. And a lot of the activities listed here are more like a treat than actual work!

For me, that's really the key when incorporating any new habit into our lives—*making it fun.* I hope this chapter showed you that movement doesn't have to be complicated or take a lot of time. You can squeeze more healthy movement into any season of life.

MOVE MORE IN ONE DAY

If you're struggling to think about when you can sneak in more movement, pull out a notebook or use a notes app to detail your entire day every 30 minutes. It might look like this:

6:30 a.m.: wake up, get ready for work
7:00 a.m.: make breakfast and coffee, make lunch, get out the door
7:30 a.m.: drive to work and settle at my desk
8:00 a.m.: team meeting
8:30 a.m.: team meeting

9:00 a.m.: bathroom break, computer work

9:30 a.m.: computer work

10:00 a.m.: phone meeting

. . . and so on.

At the end of your day, look through this list, and using the ideas from this chapter, make notes on when you can add in more movement. Is there time for a walk in the morning? Can you take the stairs instead of the elevator? Can you suggest a standing or walking meeting? Is it possible to sit on a yoga ball for part of the day? Often, it just takes a little awareness to figure out how we can become less sedentary.

30-SECOND SUMMARY

Movement is a part of life, and the more you can add to your everyday life, the better. Here are my top three strategies to rev up your metabolism, increase metabolic flexibility, and live longer with movement:

1. **Enjoy zone 2 cardio:** Exercising at a pace that allows you to hold a conversation puts you in the fat-burning zone. There are many metabolic and longevity benefits to this style of movement, and most experts agree that 150–180 minutes per week or 20–30 minutes per day will do the trick. Bonus: this comfortable pace makes it easy to do with a friend!

2. **Multitask your movement:** No one has the time to add "one more thing" to their day. You can easily stack extra movement with work calls, family activities, and house chores.

3. **Think beyond walking:** Have fun with movement by getting on the playground, pulling out your old bike, and getting down on the ground to play with your dogs. You

can also swap sitting for standing and the couch for the
floor. Yes, this counts as movement!

So far, we've covered the new, upgraded version of "diet and exercise" through managing blood sugar, building muscle, and getting in
different types of movement throughout the day. It's now time to really
go beyond the way we've approached weight loss until this point and
look at the pillars of the Metabolic Ecosystem that have just as much
impact on our appetite and weight as the foods we eat and the way we
move.

CHAPTER 5

SLEEP IS YOUR MAGIC PILL

Sleep: every living thing does it daily. You know it's important, but in relation to hunger, satiety, cravings, and metabolism, do you know *how* important? If you answered yes, do you know *why* it's so important? No matter your answers to those questions, I know you've been told that you need more sleep. But if you're like a third of Americans, you still don't make it a priority. Why?

For the same reason you don't stick to diets. "Because I said so" doesn't work on adults when the latest binge-worthy Hulu series is waiting for you or when you finally have a moment to indulgently scroll through social media at the end of the day. Once you understand how your body works, the power is in your hands: Is it worth staying up the extra hour? Does that late-night cold brew or vino trump getting quality, uninterrupted sleep? After reading this chapter, that'll be up to you to decide.

WHY DO WE NEED SLEEP?

It was only 75 years ago that scientists believed our bodies simply powered off at night. We went to sleep, things went blank, we rested, and we woke up. "But it turns out that sleep is a period during which the brain is engaged in a number of activities necessary to life—which are closely linked to quality of life," says Johns Hopkins sleep expert and neurologist Mark Wu, MD, PhD (Johns Hopkins Medicine 2021 [see "Better Sleep" in references]).

Sleep is when we renew and regenerate our system. Tissues are repaired, cells detox and turn over, and hormones—including hormones that regulate our appetite and weight—are produced and regulated. Think of sleep as a time when a janitorial team comes in and cleans up, reenergizing your body and brain to wake up fresh and ready for another day. Undersleeping disrupts this process.

Feeling tired after a poor night's sleep is a given, but you've probably also noticed feeling foggy, moody, and snacky too. Sleep is vital for the brain to retain and process information, so when we get too little of it, we tend to be forgetful and out of focus. Sleep also activates the areas in our brain that regulate emotion; without it, we struggle to handle stress. Sleep is vital to the entire body, and when we don't get enough of it, immunity is compromised, blood pressure can increase, migraines worsen, blood sugar dysregulates, and appetite increases— to name just a few consequences. But over a third of us are getting less than seven hours of sleep every night, and almost half of us are having trouble sleeping at least a few nights per week. For a species designed to be asleep and recovering for one-third of our lives, we have a serious sleep-deprivation problem.

So how much sleep do you actually need?

The American Academy of Sleep Medicine recommends a minimum of seven hours per night, and the optimal amount of sleep varies by person. Only you know how much sleep makes you feel your best. If you need help determining your ideal amount of sleep, the Rise sleep app helps you figure this out by using health data stored on your smartphone and asking a series of questions. You may find that as you start to regulate your blood sugar and reduce inflammation, your optimal amount of sleep per night will decrease. The bigger the mess, the bigger the cleanup job, so if possible, start out with as much sleep as you can get.

SLEEP AND METABOLISM

So, getting more sleep is good for you—got it. But did you know that it is also correlated with better weight management? A study conducted at the University of Chicago compared body-fat percentage with sleep duration for participants on a restricted diet. Participants lost 55 percent less body fat and 60 percent more lean tissue when they slept only 5.5 hours per night versus 8.5 hours per night. Not only that but the group who was sleep deprived experienced increased hunger. When sleep was restricted, the dieters produced higher levels of ghrelin, the hormone that triggers hunger, reduces energy expenditure, and lowers levels of our satiety hormone, leptin. Even more interesting, these participants were in a controlled environment. So, despite their increased hunger, they weren't able to satisfy that hunger with extra food. Yet, they *still* lost less body fat than the group getting adequate sleep.

Given this hormone imbalance, it's not surprising that we often feel hungrier and have increased cravings for junk food when we're sleep deprived. Brain-imaging studies show that the reward-seeking part of the brain is activated when one gets less than 7 hours of sleep per night, increasing the desire for foods that spike blood sugar and release insulin. Thus, the amount of sleep we get affects fat and muscle loss when we are trying to lose weight, and sleep deprivation makes us hangry.

A 2022 randomized clinical trial by the University of Chicago and the University of Wisconsin–Madison found that young, overweight adults who slept fewer than 6.5 hours a night consumed an average of 270 more calories per day than those who increased their sleep duration over the course of the study by 1.2 hours.

In support of this discovery, a meta-analysis found that getting less than 5.5 hours of sleep resulted in the consumption of almost 400 extra calories per day, compared with people who got more than 7 hours of sleep. Researchers also reported that the sleep-deprived individuals were more prone to food cravings and ate less protein overall.

A few more important things to know about sleep and metabolism:

1. Getting less than 5 hours of sleep increases our hunger hormone ghrelin by 15 percent and decreases our satiety hormone leptin by 15 percent. This is a perfect storm of feeling more hungry and less satiated after a night of bad sleep.

2. Resistance to insulin, the hormone that controls the amount of sugar in the blood, increases by 25 percent, resulting in increased blood sugar levels after just one night of crappy sleep! Insulin resistance is a driving factor in weight gain, weight-loss resistance, and metabolic syndrome.

3. Sleep deprivation produces higher peaks of compounds that seem to act on the same part of the brain as marijuana, making eating more pleasurable and triggering "the munchies."

4. The emotional center of the brain, the amygdala, lights up in response to highly pleasurable sugary and salty foods when we are sleep deprived, and the prefrontal cortex, which is typically responsible for making good decisions, is inhibited when we lack sleep. A double whammy!

5. Getting fewer than 6 hours of sleep while losing weight results in 55 percent less fat loss and 60 percent more lean-muscle loss than getting 8.5 hours. In other words, undersleeping while dieting will lead to a lowered BMR as it relates to muscle loss.

To sum things up, we eat more when sleep deprived, and it's *not* muscle tissue–supporting protein that we're craving. As you can see, claiming that "sleep is for the weak" is kind of like saying "water is for losers."

PAST DIETER PROFILE

No matter what Emily did, she could not drop a single pound. She worked out hard five days a week and was strict about her diet, but that workout often came at the cost of her sleep. I asked her to increase her sleep from six to seven hours per night for one week, even if that meant she would be unable to make it to the gym. She was only able to work out three times that week, instead of five, but was down two pounds by the time we met the following week. She lost weight just by working out less and sleeping more.

CIRCADIAN RHYTHM

The benefits of sleep go far beyond weight management. The amount of sleep we get at night can affect how we perform in our careers, how we show up in relationships, and our energy levels, decision-making ability, brain function, focus, self-control, blood sugar control, inflammation, food cravings, recovery time, immune system, and overall mood.

But this control center for how we show up every day isn't actually "sleep"—it's our circadian rhythm. This is the body's internal clock—a process that regulates our sleep-wake cycle. Understanding this fundamental rhythm of the body is key to understanding the importance of sleep and how to do it better.

Here is a day in the life of your circadian rhythm:

- 6:00 a.m.: Cortisol levels start to rise, and the photoreceptors in your eyes and skin turn light into electrical signals that begin to wake you up. Getting morning sunlight sets your circadian rhythm in motion and triggers the release of melatonin 12–14 hours later so that you can sleep better at night.
- 2:30 p.m.: Growth hormone and testosterone begin to rise. Until about 5:30 p.m., you'll experience a surge in these hormones that will allow you to get in your best workout. Exercising midafternoon is not possible for everyone, but if you can do it, why not?
- Sunset: As the body begins to prepare for sleep, it releases leptin and adiponectin, a potent fat-burning hormone. Our bodies are supposed to burn fat while we sleep, but we unfortunately do a lot of things that disrupt this

natural process. Both late-night eating and excessive blue light inhibit the release of these hormones at night.

- 9:00 p.m.: The body begins to release your sleepy hormone, melatonin. Melatonin turns brain activity off and gets it set to repair. However, blue light from your TV, laptop, and phone inhibits the release of melatonin. This disruption is the primary reason many people struggle with sleep.

- 12:00 a.m.: A lot of important stuff happens around midnight—but only if you're asleep. This is when fat burning, recovery, and repair from the day begin. Leptin enters the hypothalamus, and fat reserves are released. This is a vitally important process if we want to lose fat and not feel foggy the next day. The takeaway? Don't go to bed after midnight.

- 2:00 a.m.: This is when the body reaches its deepest state of sleep and goes to work on repairing damaged cells and tissues. The key to a full-body recovery from the previous day is to be asleep for a full six hours once this recovery process starts around midnight. So, again, get to bed before 12:00!

THE BLUE LIGHT-MELATONIN CONNECTION

Blue light is all around us! The sun, light bulbs, and screens all emit blue light, and the cool thing about blue light is that getting it early in the morning completely shuts down the production of melatonin (our sleep hormone), making it a natural cup of joe. The uncool thing about blue light is that, in this day and age, it's in our face constantly. Including at 10:00 p.m. while we're scrolling the socials. The blue light we encounter before going to bed is blocking melatonin production just as it does in the morning. Melatonin starts rising a few hours before bedtime, so avoiding blue light two to three hours before going to bed is the only way to not disrupt our body's natural circadian rhythm. Using blue-light blockers is essential, but if you want to really hack and optimize your sleep, use as few screens as possible in the late evening.

PRACTICE GOOD SLEEP HYGIENE

Many of us struggle with sleep for a number of reasons, but new parents, shift workers, time-zone travelers, and parents of kids who have trouble sleeping have the greatest sleep challenges. Shift workers and parents in particular are essential to our country, economy, and civilization, but they're simply not getting the quality sleep they need to perform their important jobs at the highest possible level.

Of the six players in this Metabolic Ecosystem, sleep is the one that I have historically struggled with the most. Once I discovered how important sleep is for metabolic health, I dug more deeply into the how-to research than most people would have any desire to ever do. I've tested just about every tip, hack, and device there is, and I'll share with you some of the most effective—and mostly free—sleep hacks out there.

So let's look at some solutions. The following chart highlights some common sleep problems (on the left) and ideas to try (on the right).

Trouble falling asleep	• This is likely because you're not releasing cortisol or melatonin at the appropriate times. Getting outside within a few hours of sunrise will tell your body when it's supposed to get tired at night, which will be around 10:00 p.m. (depending on what time you typically wake up). You'll want 10 minutes of sun or 30 minutes of clouds. By the way, this does not work while sitting inside your house and looking through a window. Bonus? Do the same around sundown. • Avoid caffeine 8–10 hours before bedtime—yes, this basically means coffee in the morning only. To start scaling back, have your last cup 15 minutes earlier each day until you settle on a time that doesn't seem to affect sleep. • Start dimming lights around 6:00 p.m. and have a strict no-blue-light policy after 10:00 p.m. You can use blue-light-blocking glasses with red lenses after sunset to stop the disruption of the body's release of leptin, adiponectin, and melatonin.
Waking up during the night	• Cut alcohol during the week. Alcohol doesn't actually help you fall asleep—it only sedates you. It acts on your calming neurotransmitter GABA, causing you to wake up multiple times in the night subconsciously. Alcohol also significantly disrupts REM sleep, a critical repair time for the body and brain. • Avoid light as much as possible if you're waking up anytime after 10:00 p.m., wear your blue-light blockers, and don't scroll! Advanced hack: install red lights in the bathroom you use at night.

Inconsistent sleep schedules	• Prioritize consistency as much as possible. Even if you're working the night shift only four days per week, stay as close as you can to your night-shift sleeping *and eating* schedules.
	• Sleep coach Nick Littlehales has his pro athletes count 90-minute sleep cycles, instead of total sleep, and asks them to shoot for 35 cycles per week, with a minimum of 30 cycles. It can be especially helpful for new parents to think in terms of sleep cycles when it's impossible to not have disrupted sleep.
	• A hack from my own experience—when I had my daughter, my postpartum therapist told me to focus on getting two 3-hour stretches of sleep, at a minimum, each night versus worrying about whether or not I was getting "enough sleep." This helped me structure my schedule and bedtime to ensure I'd get these 3-hour stretches, so I could feel as rested as a new mom could.

SNORING

If you feel like you're getting enough sleep, but you're still waking up in the morning feeling tired and groggy, it may be because you're snoring. Most recent statistics state that 57 percent of men and 40 percent of women snore.

There are many different reasons why we snore: nasal or sinus blockages, alcohol, smoking, medications, sleep posture, weight, and the size of our airway are some of the most common. Because snoring can disrupt sleep, it's important to first determine *why* you're snoring and then treat the issue from there. Ask a partner or roommate to observe your sleep, or set up a camera or audio device to record yourself sleeping.

If you snore

- with your mouth closed, try elevating your head four inches to encourage your tongue and jaw to move forward;
- with your mouth open, try using mouth tape (seriously, google it) to tape your mouth shut at night; this might seem absurd, but it's becoming a popular trend for a reason—mouth breathing can lead to crowded and crooked teeth, cavities, gum disease, digestive issues, chronic fatigue, and headaches;
- when sleeping on your back, try sleeping on your side;
- in all positions and your snoring is loud and heavy or if you gasp or choke in the night, get evaluated for sleep apnea.

You can start by taking the STOP-Bang Questionnaire at stopbang.ca to determine if you may have sleep apnea, and if you do, find yourself a board-certified sleep medicine doctor at sleepeducation.org.

SLEEP SUPPLEMENTS

I recommend sleep supplements with a caveat: please first fully investigate and attempt to address the underlying cause of your sleep issues. But if you are incorporating the suggestions from this chapter and want a little extra support, here are a few well-studied options. Just start with one and try it for two weeks. If it doesn't work, move on to another one. It's possible that a combination of supplements will work best for you, so be flexible until you find what works:

- theanine (200 mg): reduces stress and promotes relaxation

- ◆ magnesium bisglycinate (200 mg): relaxes the body and produces more GABA and melatonin
- ◆ magnesium threonate (145 mg): calms the central nervous
  system
- ◆ GABA (100 mg): has a calming effect on the brain and reduces anxiety
- ◆ melatonin (0.3–1.0 mg): as needed, and for short-term use
  only, to signal to the brain that it's time for sleep

30-SECOND SUMMARY

1. **Morning light:** If you do just one thing to improve your
   sleep, do this: get those eyeballs (safely) into the sun.
   Staring at your phone doesn't count, so head up! This
   habit pairs nicely with getting some movement (see chapter 4).
2. **Evening darkness:** Start flipping extra lights off around
   sunset (or 6:00 p.m. if you live in a part of the world that
   is dark most of the day). You don't have to live by candle-
   light, but any excess light you can shed in the evening will
   help.
3. **Reduce alcohol intake:** You simply can't "biohack" your
   body into being able to handle alcohol throughout the
   night. No matter what, variable blood sugar levels are
   bound to wake you up or, at the very least, cause restless
   sleep.

The weight-loss industry is still full of calorie-deficit evangelists
who will tell a client to "just eat less" even when that client claims
they're doing everything right but seeing no results. And, sure, they
might be fudging the details a bit or stuffing themselves with queso
and margs all weekend, but more often than not, there is something
deeper going on. In my years of study and working with clients, I've

found that "something deeper" is almost always one of two things: too little sleep or too much stress—or both, because the two play well together. Now that you know more about getting more (and better) sleep, let's dive into stress.

CHAPTER 6

YES, YOU CAN MANAGE YOUR STRESS!

Within an 18-month period, I went through pregnancy, postpartum, and divorce while living in a tiny, chronically flooded Atlanta apartment. I was in massive debt, was attempting to build my business, and was the sole provider for both myself and my daughter. I was undereating, overdrinking, and barely sleeping.

Even after I eventually quit drinking and started taking better care of my body, my relentless drive for success pushed me to the point of burnout and the inability to get out of bed a year later.

In that moment—when I *literally* could not get out of bed and had to call for help with my two-year-old daughter—I decided to make a radical change in the way I showed up for myself every day.

This chapter is incredibly important to me because I have been there. I am here to tell you that whether you're overwhelmed, anxious, addicted to the hustle, or chronically undernourishing yourself—or all of the above—*you don't have to keep doing it.* You've been sucked into the narrative that functioning on little sleep, relying on caffeine, and having weekly panic attacks is normal. So I'm going to talk to you how my best friend talked to me when I hit rock bottom: It's not cool. It's not admirable. And while it may be common, it's definitely not normal.

This chapter is not a list of stress-management tips. Rather, it's a look inside the human body to show how stress can break your metabolism, and then I'm going to give you the power to prevent it.

WHAT IS STRESS?

Hans Selye, the famous physiologist who first coined the term *stress*, called it "the nonspecific response of the body to any demand made upon it" (Tan and Yip 2018 [see "Stress Management" in references]).

Okay. Not super specific.

Psychologist Richard Lazarus then went a step further and called stress "an event in which biological demands, internal demands, or both, tax or exceed the adaptive resources of the individual" (Monat 1991 [see "Stress Management" in references]).

Simply put, stress is anything that taxes the body or mind.

In this chapter, we'll mostly be discussing the types of stress that *overtax* the body and mind, but it's important to point out that not all stress is "bad." A 3-minute cold plunge, a roller coaster ride, or a 100-yard sprint are all healthy "taxes" on our system. Microdosing healthy stressors can actually help us increase our resilience against what we'd consider "bad stress." But a 30-minute cold plunge, a roller coaster ride that never stops, and thirty-nine 100-yard sprints in a row would fall into the "overtaxing" category of stress.

In 2022, the American Psychological Association's Stress in America survey found that the top stressors plaguing Americans today were related to finance, relationships, loss of a loved one, loss of a job, global uncertainty, and parenting. That's all well and good, and I'm sure you recognize some of your own stressors on that list. But while your mind perceives different stressors in different ways, your body does not. The body recognizes physical stressors like undereating, overexercising, inflammation, or autoimmune disease to be in the same category as mental and emotional stressors like worrying about things that haven't happened or relationship struggles.

I don't know anyone who would say no to having less stress in their life. Aside from the obvious reasons we'd like to avoid stress—like an improved quality of life—stress has a massive impact on metabolic health. And this is where we'll be focusing our attention for this chapter. This impact is so great that every other component of the Metabolic Ecosystem falls under the umbrella of stress. Our diet, exercise regimen, sleep habits, gut health, and mindset (see chapter 8) all contribute to our body's daily stress load.

Weight gain or weight-loss resistance hits you twofold with stress. Acute stress, like rush-hour traffic or rushing your cat to the ER, might lead you to eat ice cream for dinner for that comforting dopamine hit. Chronic stress, like working a high-demand job with an asshole boss for years, can eventually lead to the downregulation of the hormonal system responsible for managing stress internally (we'll get into the details of this in a moment). Overeating after a hard day plus a dysregulated metabolic system equals a disaster for your waistline.

THE BODY'S RESPONSE TO STRESS

What really happens when our bodies are stressed? When you experience a physiological or psychological stressor, like a sweaty spin class or an argument with your partner, the information is sent to the amygdala, a part of the brain that processes memory, decision-making, and emotions. When the amygdala realizes a stressor is on deck, it sounds an alarm to the brain's command center, the hypothalamus. The hypothalamus then communicates to the adrenal glands to push out adrenaline, which prompts the body to be on high alert by increasing heart rate, sharpening focus, and releasing blood sugar and fats from storage for energy.

Once this initial surge of adrenaline subsides, the hypothalamus activates the second wave of the stress response, and cortisol is released. And once the stressor is gone, cortisol levels fall. This is the body's natural response to stress.

The problem is when stress becomes chronic, such as with ongoing financial problems, strenuous workouts seven days a week, an overly full schedule, an inflamed gut, an autoimmune disease, impossibly high expectations of oneself, uncontrolled blood sugar—this list goes on. Chronic stress means that the body's stress response remains activated all the time; cortisol and adrenaline levels don't rise and fall—they just remain elevated. This can cause damage to the blood vessels, an increased risk of heart attack and stroke, high blood sugar levels, insulin resistance, hormonal imbalances, an increase in belly fat, gut microbiome dysfunction, and increased cravings.

HOW TO MANAGE STRESS

That's a lot, I know. But our bodies were built to manage acute stress, so you don't have to eliminate every stressor in your life to feel good. You can, however, reduce the chronic stress in your life that may be causing you to cross over into metabolic distress. Let's begin by looking at a (nonexhaustive) list of common physiological and psychological stressors. Here, I'm defining *stressors* as anything that causes the adrenal glands to release excess cortisol throughout the day.

Physiological	Psychological
• poor sleep • chronic infections • inflammation • autoimmune diseases • environmental toxins • undereating • overexercising • fasting workouts • very low-carb diets • intermittent fasting • caffeine • blood sugar swings • leaky gut • food intolerances	• financial stress • marital stress • traffic • getting audited by the IRS • lack of boundaries • obsession with being busy and productive • negative self-talk • trauma • watching the news • constant stream of phone notifications • worrying about things that haven't happened • sweating the small stuff • being a parent

Now, there is nothing wrong with working through marital problems, being productive, raising kids, and drinking coffee. Everyone has a pretty high capacity for stress, because stressors are a normal part of the human experience. Think of it this way. We each have a bucket to put stressors in. If there are just a few, it's manageable; we can still carry the bucket while going about life. But we start to run into trouble when we pile too many stressors into the bucket. It gets heavier, and we have to use two hands to carry it, meaning we have less capacity to do other tasks. When the bucket starts to overflow, we have a real problem.

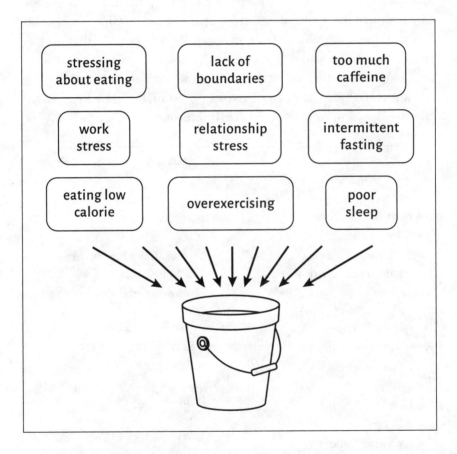

So the question becomes, How do you keep your bucket from overflowing?

1. Remove the stressors that don't need to be in the bucket.
2. Manage the stressors you can't eliminate.

Now that you're aware of what stressors may be affecting you, let's evaluate what your actual current stress load looks like. Run through the psychological and physiological stressors previously listed and write down those that resonate with you. Add any additional specific stressors that are unique to your life. This list represents your current stress bucket.

Next, cross off the "low-hanging-fruit" stressors—that is, any that are adding unnecessary stress to your life that you can easily pull out of your bucket by taking action today. Here are some examples of these kinds of stressors:

- getting less than 7 hours of sleep
- exercising on less than 7 hours of sleep
- eating less than 50 grams of carbs per day
- high-intensity workouts
- chronic long-form cardio
- intermittent fasting for more than 16 hours
- lack of boundaries
- toxic friends
- a chore you hate
- a shitty romantic partner
- the news
- doom scrolling (you know, scrolling for news that makes you believe the world is ending)
- phone notifications

I know this is easier said than done, but if you get rid of unnecessary stressors or reframe your relationship with them—which I will teach you how to do later in the chapter—you can begin to reap the benefits of lowering your stress load *immediately*.

To give you an example, let's say you are currently getting about 6 hours of sleep most nights because you're working 60 hours or more per week at your high-demand accounting job. You're up at 6:00 a.m. and out the door by 7:00 a.m., and you fast intermittently until noon. You might order an actual lunch, but you also might just snack on and off during the afternoon because you don't really have time to eat. You get home around 7:00 p.m. each night, pour a glass of wine or two, and make dinner while you snack because you're starving (and tipsy). You then get more work done until about 11:00 p.m. You lie in bed and scroll social media until about midnight.

That's a lot of stressors! Let's break it down:

- not getting enough sleep
- high-demand job
- working too many hours
- fasting
- undereating
- drinking wine in the evening
- snacking on Doritos
- lots of blue-light exposure in the evening
- scrolling
- going to bed late

What can we get rid of? You probably can't just quit your job tomorrow. But what you can do is slowly start pulling your bedtime back to 11:00 p.m., to ensure you're getting at least 7 hours of sleep. You can prep simple breakfast and lunch options for the week on Sunday so that you're no longer fasting 16 hours or more and undereating the majority of the day. You can also choose to save the wine for the weekend, as alcohol disrupts sleep quality. Perhaps set a timer so you're only scrolling for 10 minutes instead of an hour. Work boundaries are probably next on the list (can you have a chat with your manager to see about scaling back your amount of work so you don't have to get things done in the evenings?). Not only will these changes immediately lighten your stress bucket, they also will have a positive impact on blood sugar levels, energy levels, and mental clarity during your workday.

This is not a one-time exercise; I recommend reevaluating your stress bucket monthly, or even weekly. Once you get the hang of eating breakfast and lunch, cutting alcohol, and getting to bed at an earlier time, you may be able to tackle some additional stressors on your list (perhaps breaking up with a friend you've outgrown or—my personal favorite—turning off email notifications).

So then, what about the stressors you can't get rid of? You can't fix your marriage or finances with the snap of a finger; you can't control traffic during the morning commute; and some stressors—like death, moving, and a new baby—are just a normal part of life. But if you're in a particularly stressful season of life, this chapter is even more important to focus on right now. The long-term solution is to make your stress bucket bigger. You can do this by adding some tools to your toolbox to help manage the unavoidable stress in your life. You can google dozens of stress-relieving tools, but I'm going to share three high-impact tools that, through my clients, I have seen stretch the stress bucket further than you could ever imagine possible.

1. The Daily (Brain) Dump

Ever not pooped for more than a few days? It's not a good place to be physically. If you go long enough without going, you'll even end up at the doctor's office. It's normal to eliminate excess waste from our bodies every day; yet, we never think to eliminate the excess waste from our minds.

The key to the Daily (Brain) Dump is freewriting. This is not "journaling" or writing about your day in your diary—it's messy, illegible, and raw. Freewriting is often used by writers to bust through writer's block or get the creative juices flowing for the day, but you don't have to be a writer to benefit from this practice. The purpose is to remove all the popcorn popping off in your brain so that you can make room for different—and better—thoughts.

Here's what my clients have to say about the Daily (Brain) Dump:

> *This practice is my best defense at keeping anxiety at bay and getting focused on the things I want in life.*

> *I love doing this at bedtime. I let go of the day and I'm able to sleep so much better at night.*

It's a simple daily practice that can truly change your life if you let it.

Grab a notebook or journal and a pen. Set a timer for 10 minutes and pour everything in your brain onto the pages in a stream of consciousness. Sometimes it's helpful to unfocus your eyes from the page a bit, especially if you're someone who has a hard time getting messy.

Do not—I repeat—do not be tempted to write legibly. You have to be able to keep up with your running thoughts as you do this. You should not be able to read your writing easily, and the words you're putting to paper don't have to make sense. Just write whatever comes to mind, even if it's "stupid"—no one is going to be able to read it!

This will feel awkward at first, and you won't have a clue what to write about. Your first entry might look like:

> *I have no idea what I'm even writing about this is so stupid why am I doing this Megan is crazy I'm so stressed right now I don't even have the time to be doing this honestly if I just strapped on some balls and quit my job . . .*

You can google "journal prompts" and find thousands. But when you're first starting out, I'm challenging you to write without prompts. This is an important exercise in letting go, and part of that is letting go of expectations about what to write every day. There are no expectations here. Just put the pen to paper and go!

Do this practice daily, or three days a week at a minimum.

2. Flip the Script

In June of 2020, I had just become a single mom and was struggling financially during the pandemic—with a newborn. I was terrified and had no clue what I was going to do next. Knowing I needed help, a good friend sent me a podcast that would change my life forever: the *Life Coach School Podcast* with Brooke Castillo. Castillo's "The Model" teaches that thoughts produce feelings, feelings fuel actions, and actions create results. And most importantly, thoughts are *not* circumstances. Whoa.

For example, my life being an absolute shit show was actually not my current circumstance—it was a thought inside my head. Castillo taught me that the drama inside my head can only be considered a circumstance if it can be proved in a court of law. Otherwise, it's just a thought. And you can change your thoughts.

I've simplified the model for myself—and for you—to flipping the script. I'll give you a real-life example of how this has worked in my own life.

Thought: *I'm never going to get this book written with all these appointments this week!*

This thought set off a normal, healthy stress response in my body. I felt panic, overwhelmed, and resentment toward being a single parent who has to handle everything. I could feel the adrenaline start to pump and cortisol start to rise. But because I'm in the habit of using this tool, I stopped myself, realized that *I'm never going to get this book written* was only a thought and not a circumstance, and I flipped the script.

Flip the script: *The appointment with my CPA will save me money in taxes, the appointment with my financial planner will prepare me for my dream retirement on my party yacht, and the podcast I have scheduled to record will help spread my message to new people. I'm busy, but this is an exciting season of growth.*

Wow, doesn't that feel nice? Let's try a few more:

Thought: *I feel fat.*

Flip the script: *My clothes are not comfortable today.*

Thought: *I hate laundry.*

Flip the script: *Laundry is a great time to call my mom and catch up.*

Thought: *I'm never going to lose this weight.*

Flip the script: *I've done many things in my life that I never thought possible, and this is no different.*

But you don't have to take my word for it. Put it to the test—right now! List three different thoughts floating around in your head that are adding stress to your life. It could be something major like finances or minor like not having the energy to make dinner for your family tonight. Then flip the script!

Here is the most important part of this exercise: notice the difference in what you feel, the sensations in your body when writing out or reading the revised thought. That magic is why this is one of my top three rules for a less stressed life.

Make this a daily practice. Write down one to three thoughts each morning or night and flip the script. The more you practice, the more you'll begin to do this automatically in your head throughout the day.

3. Breath Work

Breath work has been used in Chinese, Japanese, and Indian traditions for thousands of years, both therapeutically and as a path to spiritual awakening. Breath work can be defined as any technique that guides you to intentionally control the way you breathe. It is often used as a stress reduction tool that brings both mental and physical relaxation.

In a study conducted at the University of Arizona, participants were asked to use either breath work or more-conventional, cognitive strategies such as reframing your stress (or, flipping the script!) for stress management. Those in the breath work group not only showed more benefits in terms of stress and mood management in the moment but also felt greater effects even three months later.

How does one measure stress levels objectively? Well, participants were asked to experience a high-pressure situation while their breathing and heart rate were measured. The group who practiced breath work maintained a steady breath and heart rate prior to the high-stress situation, while the others did not. What researchers concluded from these results was that breath work had created a buffer against anxiety in what would normally be an anxiety-producing situation.

So, why is simply focusing on intentional breathing more effective than "minding your mind" on its own? When we are stressed, our prefrontal cortex—the decision-making, rational part of the brain—becomes impaired. And at that point, it can be difficult to simply talk yourself out of a reaction. Changing the rhythm of your breath, on the other hand, creates physiological changes in the body that can signal a state of relaxation. It slows your heart rate and activates the parasympathetic nervous system, which is responsible for keeping us in a calm state. You breathe, your body slows down, you connect back to the present moment, and your ability to be rational returns.

I like to think of breath work as a form of active meditation. If you struggle with the concept of sitting still and quieting your mind, breath work is like a hack: you sit still and focus on your breath, which has the added bonus of quieting your mind!

To get started on utilizing this technique for managing stress, pull out your phone and set your alarm to go off every hour tomorrow with a reminder to stop and breathe. While counting to four, take a deep, slow breath; then count to four again as you let it out. Do this a few times.

This subtle reminder throughout the day will bring you right back to where you belong—in the present moment! Unless you're in immediate danger, the present moment is almost never a scary place. We create so much fear and anxiety by thinking about what's already happened and how it might affect our future. Once you get a little more comfortable becoming aware of your breath, you can dip your toes into the actual practice of breath work.

There are many forms of breath work, and I encourage you to explore this world and find a practice that works for you. The type of breath work that I have personally found to consistently calm my nervous system, give me clarity, and boost my creativity is intermittent hypoxia training (IHT), which uses breath retention (in other words, holding your breath) to build up CO_2, help the body adapt to lower levels of oxygen, and prevent oxidative stress. Putting your body into a purposeful, safe state of stress like this, while remaining cool, calm, and collected, increases your capacity for stress in real life. SOMA Breath and the Wim Hof Method are two types of IHT breath work that I use daily, and you can try out each of these breath techniques on the SOMA Breath or Wim Hof YouTube channels. I like to switch it up, depending on my mood!

You can practice breath work daily or even just a few times per week to benefit.

30-SECOND SUMMARY

While you cannot always control the circumstances in your life, you can always control the way you think about those circumstances. This chapter offers tools to know which stressors you can remove from your stress bucket to lighten the load, and how to make that bucket a bit bigger for this particular season.

Prioritize sleep above all else. Exercise, but be mindful of whether or not that exercise is adding to your stress load or supporting it. Eat to balance your blood sugar. Pay attention to digestion—it tells you a lot about how your nervous system is functioning. Walk in the sunshine. And you probably need therapy, so, if possible, do that too. You've got this.

1. **Stress is a leading cause of weight-loss resistance.**
    It includes physical stress such as overexercising or

undereating, psychological stress such as marital or financial stress, and internal stress such as a chronic disease or an autoimmune disease.

2. **Decrease your stress load** whenever possible by removing the controllable stressors from your life, like too much caffeine, overexercising, and fasting for more than 12 hours.

3. **Increase your capacity for stress** by keeping a regular hygiene practice of freewriting, flipping the script, and more-intentional breathing.

As you start to make these changes in the way you eat, move, sleep, and manage stress, you will no doubt start to feel the difference in your body immediately. But when we dive into the final element of the Metabolic Ecosystem, a healthy gut, we're going to talk about something that can be difficult to quantify—inflammation. While it is a leading cause of weight-loss resistance, most of us have no idea that inflammation is lurking in our system.

CHAPTER 7

GUT CHECK

We need to talk about your gastrointestinal (GI) tract.

We can't have a discussion about metabolism without discussing inflammation, and we can't have a discussion about inflammation without discussing the state of the tube that runs from your mouth to your anus—also known as your gut. A healthy gut is the sixth and final piece of the Metabolic Ecosystem pie.

But before we really dive in, understand that this chapter is nowhere near a comprehensive guide to gut health. There could be an entire encyclopedia written on this topic. Our gut microbiome consists of the microorganisms that inhabit the digestive tract, and it has an impact on nearly every system in the human body. (If you're interested in learning more about this, check out the resources section.) For the purposes of this book, I will stick to how the gut affects our metabolic health and what you can do to make sure you're protecting it. My goal is both to bring awareness to the role of the gut in this ecosystem and to give you the immediate tools to address this silent metabolism killer.

WHAT IS GUT HEALTH?

The term *gut health* refers to the function and balance of the bacteria that populate the GI tract. In this chapter, I'll use the terms *bacteria*, *microbes*, or *microbiota*, and these are interchangeable. I'm simply referring to the little critters that line the elaborate tube that runs through our bodies, starting at the mouth and ending at the anus. I know, thinking about your body being lined with bacteria doesn't sound like a good thing, but these microbes have the power to affect nearly every aspect of your health, including your digestion, how your brain and body respond to stress, your immune system, inflammation, and much, much more.

I like to think of the gut as the place where the outside world meets our inside world; everything we ingest takes a ride on the microbial gut train. This is where food is broken down, metabolized, absorbed, and utilized or eliminated.

But the gut is so much more than a pathway for sustenance throughout the body. The microbiota in our gut release chemicals as they interact with the food we eat, and these chemicals carry out some pretty important jobs, such as regulating 75–80 percent of our immune system, controlling our metabolism, and communicating with our brain and organs. Basically, the more scientists and researchers learn about this complex system, the more they realize that our microbiota have an impact on nearly every aspect of our being, which includes our ability to manage our weight.

Because so many other body systems are reliant on a functioning GI tract, you can start to see why the rest of the body can easily be thrown off when something is off in the gut. And the main culprit of issues in the gut is inflammation.

Inflammation is an incredibly important and protective response to something the body doesn't like, such as a germ, an infection, or an injury. Inflammation's job is to bring more immune cells to the affected part of the body so that the healing process can begin. But when the body isn't able to fully heal, it remains inflamed, which can lead to chronic fatigue, chronic pain, depression, anxiety, a lowered immune system, digestive problems, and weight-loss resistance.

When it comes to inflammation in the gut, the number one culprit is too much "bad" bacteria. The inflammation occurs on the gut lining, which serves as a wall that dictates what gets in and what gets out. When the lining becomes repeatedly inflamed, it can start to break down and become permeable, or "leaky," as it is often called.

So now, instead of serving as a barrier between the gut and the rest of your body, the leaky gut lining can allow toxins, bacteria, and partially digested food particles into the bloodstream. When this happens, the body has another inflammatory response against the foreign invaders. Inflammation in the gut can often lead to larger, systemic inflammation throughout the whole body, and that's bad news on several fronts:

1. When your body is constantly putting out an inflammation fire, fat burning is deprioritized so that the body can focus on cooling the inflammation. And if this is a round-the-clock job, it makes weight loss impossible.
2. An inflamed gut can have an impact on our mental health: 95 percent of serotonin, which plays a key role in mood, sleep, and digestion, is made in the gut. An imbalance in the gut can lead to poor serotonin production, thereby negatively affecting sleep, mood regulation, and gut motility.
3. Worldwide, three out of five people die because of chronic inflammatory diseases like stroke, heart disease, cancer, obesity, respiratory diseases, or diabetes, which is why inflammation prevention has become such a hot—and vital—topic in the health-care field.
4. Inflammation is a tax on the body, making chronic inflammation an *overtax*. Chronic inflammation is a big stressor, and one that you'll want to work toward removing from your stress bucket.

Let's say you know you have a gluten intolerance, but you eat the bread anyway because "it's so worth it!" When you ingest something that the body recognizes as a foreign invader (in this case, a piece of bread), the blood vessels in the digestive tract enlarge and become more permeable, which brings more white blood cells to the site of the injury. An inflammatory response occurs just as if you had cut your finger. Within 12–15 hours after the offending food is consumed, immune activity stops and the gut begins the healing process, which can take months—and that's only if there is no more exposure to that food. But if you continue to eat the offending food, the inflammatory response just repeats and repeats itself until, eventually, that cell lining will start to break down.

But it's not just food intolerances that trigger inflammation in the gut. As a matter of fact, food intolerances are often just a byproduct of existing microbial imbalances! The following is a nonexhaustive list of ways that the gut microbiome can become imbalanced and eventually inflamed:

- artificial sweeteners
- chronic infections from viruses, bacteria, fungi, or parasites
- chronic stress
- environmental toxins
- low stomach acid
- medications like hormonal birth control, NSAIDs (non-steroidal anti-inflammatory drugs), and PPIs (proton-pump inhibitors)
- nervous system dysregulation
- nutrient deficiencies
- poor sleep
- processed foods
- repeated antibiotic use

What might you experience with an inflamed gut? Here is another nonexhaustive list of some of the common symptoms:

- anxiety or depression
- acne, psoriasis, eczema, or rashes
- ADHD (attention deficit hyperactivity disorder)
- autoimmune disease
- bad breath
- digestive issues (diarrhea, constipation, heartburn, and acid indigestion)
- fatigue/brain fog
- food intolerances or sensitivities
- gas/bloating

- heart disease
- joint pain/muscle aches
- poor immune function
- seasonal allergies
- trouble sleeping
- weight-loss resistance/weight gain

MANAGE YOUR MICROBIOME

So, clearly, gut health needs to be a priority, whether you're looking to lose weight, feel better, live longer, or all of the above. The three most common quick wins I see when implementing some of the tools from this chapter are improved digestion, a reduction in bloating, and clearer skin.

The good news is that even when gut inflammation or an imbalance is suspected, you can often explore healing at home. To begin, eat high-quality, nutrient-dense proteins, healthy fats, and fiber-rich carbs that balance blood sugar; stay hydrated; incorporate electrolytes; don't overdo it at the gym; move your body every day; get quality sleep; and manage your stress.

If no improvements in symptoms are seen in four months, I recommend working with a functional-nutrition dietitian or another functional-health-care provider. You may need a gut mapping or additional labs to take a deeper look at what's going on.

You are your microbiome. Your microbiome is you. That said, your microbiome is not your destiny. Often, simply nourishing yourself and emptying your stress bucket will clear up a lot of your gut issues over time. And if it doesn't, remember that there are so many resources dedicated to healing the gut.

Supporting the gut comes down to three steps:

1. **Cut** out anything that causes an imbalance in the microbiome.
2. **Heal** any damage that has been done.
3. **Feed** the gut with foods it needs to thrive.

Cut

Your first line of defense against a bad gut is limiting processed foods in your diet. In other words, choose more whole foods over processed foods. The reasons for this are numerous, but simply put, our body's microbiome evolved to prefer whole foods like vegetables, fruits, and meats, not frozen chicken nuggets and boxed cereal. There are plenty of books written on this topic if you want to go deeper (see the resources section), but here are a few specific foods to look out for.

Check your frozen and pantry foods for oils like canola, cottonseed, vegetable, sunflower, safflower, corn, and soybean, and slowly start to swap these inflammatory oils for coconut, avocado, and sustainable palm oils. Skip items with artificial sweeteners, flavors, and colors, as well as anything with high-fructose corn syrup, soy protein, or soy flour. There are plenty of other ingredients to avoid, but these are some of the most common ingredients in highly processed foods. Also, don't shoot the messenger, but alcohol has been shown to negatively affect the microbiome. In the end, though, this isn't about being perfect. It's about awareness and making swaps when you can.

If you're making swaps and still having symptoms of poor gut health, you may be intolerant or sensitive to something you're eating, or your body may not be producing enough of the enzymes needed to break down certain foods—even if those foods are "healthy"! Any type of food can cause inflammatory reactions in your body when it's already struggling with damage in the gut. Raw vegetables, chia seeds, nuts, and eggs are a few of the most common, because they are more difficult for the body to digest. You may need to remove these foods if they are causing you problems (although see "Heal" for an alternative solution) and then get to work on repairing your gut before adding them back.

PAST DIETER PROFILE

Michelle was eating PHFF at every meal, strength training three or four times a week, and sleeping well after working with me for several weeks. She felt good but was frustrated at the lack of physical changes.

Every day around 2:00 p.m., Michelle started to bloat, and by the time she went to bed, she described herself as looking "six months pregnant." I noticed she was eating green peppers every day at lunch, so I had her cut them out for a couple of weeks. By our next session, she had lost 6 pounds. It turned out that Michelle was intolerant to "nightshade vegetables" like peppers, tomatoes, and eggplant. We removed the green peppers from her diet and started a gut-healing protocol, and her weight loss continued over the next few months until she was down 15 pounds.

Heal

Removing what's causing the damage is a vital first step in supporting the gut, but healing the damage that's already been done is often skipped. Along with using the following strategies to help heal the gut, I love utilizing them after a round of antibiotics or a bout of diarrhea or food poisoning to get things back on track:

- glutamine: 3 grams per day between meals
- bone broth/bone-broth powder: 1–2 cups bone broth per day or one serving of bone-broth powder
- gelatin: one serving per day
- sleep: seven hours or more per night (because sleep is when the body heals!)

While you may not be able to digest certain foods because your body has become intolerant, it's also possible that you're just underproducing the stomach acid and digestive enzymes needed to digest those foods. You have to be able to break down and metabolize the food you're eating! Three big red flags for improper digestion are acid indigestion, upset stomach, and bloating, and there's an easy test you can do at home to see if your stomach acid is low (see sidebar).

DO I HAVE LOW STOMACH ACID?

Let's find out. First thing in the morning, mix 1/4 teaspoon of baking soda in 6 ounces of water and drink it on an empty stomach. If you burp within three minutes, you probably have sufficient stomach acid. If you don't burp or it takes longer than three minutes, you probably have low stomach acid.

If you are dealing with these red flags, here is a list of strategies I recommend trying:

- Digestive bitters: While taking digestive-enzyme supplements can be helpful in the short term, digestive bitters can actually help the body start to produce more enzymes and acid on its own. Fair warning: this doesn't taste like candy!
- Apple cider vinegar: I don't like this as well as digestive bitters, but if you have it around the house, you could add 1–2 teaspoons of apple cider vinegar to 2–3 tablespoons of water and drink prior to meals.
- Chew your food: Maybe it's a lack of digestive enzymes, but it could also be the fact that you're inhaling your food over a sink between calls. Make it a habit to chew your food to an applesauce consistency before swallowing and watch bloat disappear. As a bonus, chewing food more thoroughly gives your body time to send satiety signals that will stop you from overeating.

- Cook your veggies: Can't digest raw veggies? No need to force a salad down. Just lightly cook or steam your vegetables and see if that helps.
- Marinate meats: Prepare meats in an acid, like lemon juice or vinegar, and use a pressure cooker to really break down muscle fibers, for easy digestion.
- Fast for 10–12 hours: Your digestive system is like I-285 in metro Atlanta at 5:00 p.m. (i.e., it's *really* busy!). If you don't give it a break every once in a while, you'll eventually end up gridlocked. Give it a rest by not consuming calories from after dinner until breakfast the next morning.

Feed

Supporting your gut is a lifelong practice—it's not one and done! If you stop exercising, you will slowly lose the benefits of exercise. In the same way, if you heal your gut only to stop eating gut-supportive foods, you will start to create an imbalance in healthy and unhealthy bacteria.

As mentioned in the "Cut" section, whole foods are the way to go, as they are more nutrient dense and contain fewer inflammatory ingredients than processed foods. A great rule of thumb for a happy gut is to simply eat more plant-based foods. There is more than enough data to advise us all to live by Michael Pollan's popular advice from his book *In Defense of Food*: "Eat food. Not too much. Mostly plants." And that is coming from 50 years of clear clinical nutrition research. In addition, eating a variety of foods is key. The more diverse your diet, the more diverse the bacteria in your gut will be. A sparsely diverse microbiome is linked to inflammation and a leaky gut. Here are a couple of other tips to try as you continue on your gut-health journey, but keep in mind that, unfortunately, popping a supplement every day, thinking you're healing your gut, is not the easy way out.

1. Probiotics are the healthy bacteria that populate your gut.
    •   Include fermented foods like sauerkraut, kimchi, raw
        pickles, kombucha, raw dairy products, homemade
        sourdough bread, miso, and tempeh.
    •   Take a high-quality spore-based probiotic supplement
        like Just Thrive.
2. Prebiotics are what probiotics in your body feed on to
    multiply and grow.
    •   Eat more fiber. Get a variety of fruits, vegetables,
        starchy carbs, beans, legumes, nuts, and seeds. If
        grains, nuts, or seeds bother your stomach, try soaking
        or sprouting them first.
    •   Add acacia fiber, psyllium husk, or partially hydrolyzed
        guar gum to coffee or tea or sprinkle over foods for
        extra prebiotic fiber.

30-SECOND SUMMARY

A healthy microbiome population in the gut communicates with cells
all over the body and can affect your nervous system, your immune system, your digestive system, your mental health, and your metabolism.

1. An unhealthy gut triggers chronic inflammation, which is
    one of the primary sources of weight-loss resistance.
2. To reduce inflammation in the gut, cut anything causing
    damage, heal any damage that has already been done, and
    feed the gut with the foods it needs to thrive.
3. Making sure the body can absorb the food and nutrients
    you are consuming is vital to healing the gut. Using diges-
    tive bitters; chewing your food; lightly cooking vegetables;
    soaking grains, seeds, and nuts; and giving your digestive
    system a break by fasting for 10–12 hours are some simple
    ways to prep the body to absorb the nutrients it needs to
    restore gut health.

Over these last six chapters, you've learned about the Metabolic Ecosystem—blood sugar control, muscle, movement, sleep, stress management, and a healthy gut. Together, these pillars will enable you to move beyond a power struggle with food and tap into your body and how it really works. I hope you can now understand that your body is not the enemy and that it actually wants to support you properly. This whole system works together to optimize hormones, regulate hunger, and rev up your metabolism. You were born with the ability to regulate your body weight, and with these tools, you can absolutely get that ability back.

Now, it's time to take what you've learned and integrate it into your real life.

CHAPTER 8

TRAIN YOUR BRAIN

Now that you have all the details on each of the six pillars that make up the Metabolic Ecosystem, it's time I let you in on a little secret. If we zoom out and take a ten-thousand-foot view, the Metabolic Ecosystem in its entirety is only 20 percent of losing weight, keeping it off, and never going on another diet again.

The other 80 percent is right inside your head.

THE POWER OF THE SUBCONSCIOUS MIND

The mind is perhaps the most mysterious part of the human being. Sure, we know about the brain as an organ, its structure and how it works like a computer, processing information through chemical and electrical signals. But the mind—that's a place you can't really map. In fact, it's not really a place at all; it's more of a collection of experiences, synonymous with our thoughts, emotions, memories, and beliefs. And there is still a lot we don't know about this crucial component of what makes us human.

What we do know is that there are two components of our mind—the conscious and subconscious—that dictate our thoughts, actions, and experiences daily. The conscious mind is anything we are aware of in the current moment: what we are feeling, doing, touching, saying, and experiencing. The subconscious mind, on the other hand, contains all the information from our past experiences. It affects the way we feel and how we respond, react, and experience life. According to psychologist Benjamin Hardy, "what happens on your subconscious level influences what happens on your conscious level. In other words, what goes on internally, even subconsciously, eventually becomes your reality" (Hardy 2021 [see "Mindset" in references]).

Neuroscientists have agreed for years, and recent science proves, that the majority of our thoughts and, therefore, corresponding actions come from our subconscious mind.

Let's look at a couple of real-life examples of the conscious and subconscious minds in action. Consider someone who decides to start riding a bike for the first time in 15 years. She has no recollection of her first bike lesson as a child, but she hops on and effortlessly takes off. Her subconscious mind has stored all the information she needs to ride a bike, and her conscious mind can pay attention to stop signs and curbs. This is an example of our subconscious mind stepping up and making life easier for us.

Next, consider someone who has hit snooze every morning for the past 15 years. When he decides he wants to start jumping out of bed at the crack of dawn, it only lasts a few days before he's hitting snooze again. Sound familiar? He's quick to blame that lack of follow-through on willpower, but the reality is that, for the past 15 years, his subconscious mind has been in control. He is programmed to hit the snooze button the second his alarm goes off because that decision stopped being conscious a long time ago. This is an example of our subconscious mind having an agenda based on a past experience that is in conflict with a goal we set in our conscious mind.

A slightly different example of this is the famous Good Samaritan experiment done at Princeton University. A group of divinity students were to deliver a sermon in their next class, but the researchers purposely made them late and planted a person who appeared distressed in the hallway outside their classroom. Despite these students' values, their goal to get to class on time overrode their moral obligation to help a person in need, and the majority did not stop to help. Researchers concluded that "conflict, rather than callousness," explained their failure to stop (Darley and Batson 1973 [see "Mindset" in references]).

The point is that, despite our values, we may have some other goal that conflicts with our intentions. And if the habit we're trying to change is not as perceivably important as another conflicting goal that's operating at the subconscious level, our conscious mind does a wonderful job of coming up with excuses to help us avoid changing.

So how do we influence our subconscious mind to get on board with our desire to become a morning person (or, you know, eat more vegetables, get to the gym four days per week, or drop the daily wine habit)?

LOGICAL LEVELS

The answer is to go from wanting to change your life to *deciding* to change your life. When I was first introduced to Robert Dilts's Logical Levels model, I realized this was exactly how one does just that. Not only has this model shaped the way I've approached deciding to change my own life, it is now an integral part of the way I coach clients. It offers a framework for lasting change beyond temporary or situational behavior modification.

The model applies an understanding of neurology to explain how we create change in our lives and suggests that change occurs in a hierarchy of mutually influencing levels, as shown in the following chart. These levels offer insight into how our thoughts, actions, and results are all connected. According to Dilts, "the function of each level is to synthesize, organize and direct the interactions on the level below it. . . . Meaning, when change occurs on a higher level, permanent behavior change is far more likely to occur" (Oakwater 2018 [see "Mindset" in references]). For example, the diet industry asks us to make changes on the bottom two levels of the pyramid—the environment and behavior levels. It asks us to change our environment by joining a gym and cleaning out our pantries, and it asks us to change our behavior by eating less and exercising more. But without traveling further up the pyramid, permanent behavior—and permanent weight loss—is far less likely to occur. Let's take a closer look at each of the levels to discover what this could look like for you.

PURPOSE

IDENTITY

BELIEFS

CAPABILITIES

BEHAVIORS

ENVIRONMENT

Environment: The Where

When we think of changing our behaviors around diet and exercise, we often think about the place or location involved in making this change: *I'm going to join a gym so I can restart my exercise habit.* At this level, behavior change is seen through the lens of location—home, work, the gym, a restaurant, a hotel—anywhere that you are making decisions about food and your body. Environments can often influence how you react to a stimulus.

For example, how is your environment supporting the decisions you're making? Is your kitchen filled with foods that support your goals? When you go out to eat, do you choose restaurants that make you feel good? Do you love your gym or do you dread going to it?

We make decisions about our environment on a conscious level, so what are some conscious decisions you can make to change your environment to make decision-making easier? This might include removing foods from the house that are not in alignment with how you want to feel—which also might include a conversation with your partner or kids about your goal. Perhaps it includes finding a place to exercise that makes you feel good and welcome—a place you *want* to go to!

Behaviors: The What

This level refers to your actions within an environment. Typically, the goal of a behavior is to reach a desired outcome, and our behaviors tend to dominate our action plan toward our goals. Some behavior changes you may have made so far just by reading this book might include eating PHFF at every meal, incorporating strength training a few times a week, and prioritizing a morning walk.

When you think about your current behaviors, how are they supporting your goal?

This is the level where we tend to stop when working toward a goal. But as you learned with the example of the divinity students at the beginning of the chapter, habit change can be difficult when there is another goal (indulging in a true-crime docuseries marathon) that conflicts with your new intentions (getting eight hours of sleep). Your conscious mind excels at coming up with rationalizations, and willpower cannot override the subconscious when it's found a better reason to stay up late than to go to bed.

Capabilities: The How

This level refers to the plans, strategies, and skills you acquire to create change and help guide your behaviors within your environment. They direct the decisions that you make, whether conscious or subconscious.

As you are reading this book, you are creating change at the capability level. What you now understand about food and your body is generating different behaviors directed within your environment. Instead of following a particular diet and exercise plan (behavior level), you're now making daily decisions for yourself based on what you've learned.

What makes decision-making at the capability level easier as you acquire new information is that you come into a new awareness as to why you might want to make a different decision. When I first began to question the diet industry mantra of "eat less and exercise more," I had been hearing that weight lifting could be a more effective weight-loss strategy than daily cardio. But I didn't decide to actually give it a shot until I had read an article that explained why. The science and logic I learned helped override my fear of dropping calorie-burning cardio from my routine and trying something different. That doesn't mean you can't use a meal plan or hire a trainer—it just means that you're lifting weights now in response to a new awareness and under-standing of what lean-muscle mass does for your metabolic rate and body composition, not because Trainer Brad told you to.

Beliefs: The Why

This level provides the driving force that either supports or inhibits your environment, behaviors, and capabilities. Beliefs are *why* you fol-low through (or don't) on a course of action to create change.

We often act based on what we believe to be true about ourselves, based on previous experiences. So, if your experience is *I self-sabotage* and *I've hated how I look in shorts since 2008* and that is what you be-lieve, it will become difficult to continue to utilize your knowledge of the Metabolic Ecosystem after the initial excitement phase wears off. These *limiting beliefs* put a ceiling on what you believe you're capa-ble of.

Beliefs are a little like weeds. Sometimes they're easy to pull, and it's just a matter of recognizing them and bringing them into the light. Other times they have deep roots, and it can take a lot of self-reflection and self-work to pull them out. Some of my favorite healing modali-ties for overcoming these deep-seated beliefs are therapy, inner-child work, and the Emotional Freedom Technique/tapping (you can find out more about these in the resources section).

However, the exercise toward the end of this chapter is a powerful first step in recognizing your limiting beliefs. Bringing these beliefs into the light can often be the catalyst you need to begin to change them.

Identity: The Who

Ah, my personal favorite! This level refers to who you are and demonstrates your self-worth. This is who you are at an "I am" level. I am an author. I am a morning person. I am someone who prioritizes my energy every day.

One way to bust through the limiting beliefs you may have about yourself is by changing your identity. I know, so simple, right? But because your beliefs are so ingrained and influenced by your past, sometimes changing who you are can actually be a simpler process.

You can think of your identity change as a rebrand. Cindy Kemp, one of my clients, introduced this concept to me, and I've been using it with other clients ever since. Think of yourself as you are today, and then think of yourself as the person you desire to be, achieving the goals you desire to achieve, a year from now. Those are *not* the same two people! If you are the same version of yourself a year from now, you will not have achieved the goals you set for yourself. So, what does that new version of yourself look like? What's *on-brand* for the new you?

For example, when Cindy made the decision to feel good every day (this was her goal), she knew she couldn't continue living in a constant binge-restrict cycle, drinking multiple nights per week, and allowing the scale to dictate a good or bad day. Using "I am" statements, Cindy's rebrand looked like this:

1. I am a person who gets back on track immediately. If I decide to enjoy dessert or nachos at a baseball game, I simply return to eating PHFF at the next meal, and I don't turn a treat into a binge fest.
2. I am never hungover.
3. I am a person who wears fun, bold earrings because I am a fun, bold person.
4. I am a person who goes to live concerts—often.
5. I am a person who does not step on the scale.
6. I am a person who exercises four days per week. No matter what. Even if it's for 10 minutes.

Take it from Cindy herself:

> *I've done every diet you could possibly imagine in the last 15 years. One year ago today, I made the decision that I was done disrespecting myself. I became a person who gave herself grace, who didn't step on the scale anymore, and who loved the body she was in today, tomorrow, and a year from now. I'm down 25 pounds, I'm nicer to my husband, and I talk to myself like I talk to my best friend. They say you can't change overnight, but you can when you decide to.*

When you decide that you are a person who is never hungover, you are no longer just telling yourself to quit drinking so much. If you're a person who never gets hungover and that's a part of your identity, you will put more focus on doing things that prevent a hangover, rather than simply attempting to use willpower to drink less. For example, you might research ways to mitigate a hangover, read a book about quitting alcohol, or get an accountability partner who also wants to scale back on drinking.

Purpose: Life Goals

This level refers to your overall mission and goals in life. Think of this level as your "higher purpose" or the spiritual force that guides and shapes your life.

Think about how your goal fits into your higher purpose. It may feel a little ridiculous to have a spiritual connection with wanting to feel confident in a pair of shorts next summer, but perhaps you just need to reframe the way you're thinking about it. Perhaps living in a healthy body you love contributes to your confidence in living out your life of purpose.

Making change on the purpose level can feel a little esoteric and hard to pin down, so I prefer to work mostly on the identity level. But it can certainly be helpful to understand how your goal fits into your larger vision.

EXPLORE YOUR LOGICAL LEVELS

To close this chapter, I have an exercise I'd like you to complete. Please do not skip this. You can read the final chapter first if you'd like, but if you want the pages of this book to be worthwhile, you'll come right back here.

Make the decision that you are now the type of person who doesn't give up on themselves. You don't stop. When you have a bad-body-image day or you step on the scale and hate what it says, you no longer throw in the towel. You are now the 2.0 version of yourself—full stop— and quitting on yourself is no longer an option.

My dream for you as you complete this exercise and move forward with implementing what you've learned in this book is that you will discover what it feels like to fall in love with taking care of yourself. When you focus on feeling as good as hell and let go of the expectations you've put on yourself, your entire life opens up.

Setup

Choose a goal you have for yourself over the next 12 months. This could be related to your body, health, finances, family, living situation, relationships—anything. For example, *I want to feel sexy and confident in my clothes.*

Steps

1. Environment: Make a list of your common environments; then write down how each makes you feel and how they affect your decision-making. If there are environments that you feel cause you to make decisions that are not in alignment with your goal, how can you change them? Create an action plan to make changes within your specific environments.

2. Behaviors: We repeat most of the same habits and behaviors every day, so walk through your day and write down your common behaviors—starting with when your alarm goes off in the morning to when you go to bed. For each behavior, place a checkmark next to those that are supporting your goal and an *X* next to those that are not. Do not do anything else with this list for now.

3. Capabilities: You're already beginning the work by reading this book! Look at your behaviors list and note some of the behaviors you're not so thrilled about: Are there any other resources you can tap into to help you learn more about change in those areas? Perhaps a book or podcast about sleep, mindset, or gut health? Have you been thinking about working with someone on your digestive issues but haven't pulled the trigger? Are you feeling unconfident in the gym and need to hire a trainer to help? Make sure to check the resources section for some of my recommendations.

4. Beliefs: Write down your goal on the top of a new page; you're going to do some journaling, using these questions as a starting point: What about this goal feels uncomfortable to you? What do you believe to be true about reaching this goal within this time frame? Why do you hold these beliefs? Is the reason due to something that happened in the past? Something in your childhood? Spend 15 minutes—or however long you like—writing on these questions and then move on. We'll come back to this.

5. Identity: Spend some time visualizing yourself a year from now, having accomplished your goal. How do you feel every day? What are you wearing? What time do you wake up? What do your relationships look like? What do you do for fun? Then make your rebrand list. Use present-tense statements, such as:

- I am a person who works out three or four times a week.
- I am full of energy.
- I am a person who feels hot and confident in their clothes.
- I am assertive with my wants and needs.

6. Purpose: Think about the final decade of your life. How do you want to feel? What do you want to be doing? When you reflect back on your life, what are you most proud of accomplishing? How does your goal fit into this overall vision?

PAST DIETER PROFILE

Kaitlin was a part of the Metabolism Makeover community for a year and still had not lost any weight. She worked 12–14-hour days and admitted she constantly put herself last. After doing a training in the community on the levels of change, she made the decision that she was no longer a person who gave up on herself and she went all in. For the first time in Kaitlin's life, she figured out what made her feel good every day—and she did it. Kaitlin began losing inches almost immediately after making this decision and hasn't stopped putting herself first ever since.

YOUR NEW LIFE CAN START TODAY

You might have come out of that exercise feeling invigorated and inspired to make the decision to start your new life. Or, instead, that exercise might have made you feel frustrated, stuck, or even triggered.

If you felt frustrated because it was impossible to think ahead two weeks, let alone one year, it may be because you've been living unintentionally for so long that you don't have a clue how to make that shift into more-intentional living. You are not alone. As a matter of fact, I see this with clients all the time! I highly recommend the Daily (Brain) Dump practice in chapter 6 to begin to clear the popcorn out of your brain and start making more room for what you really want in this life. I've seen this practice be really effective for those who are in your shoes. Practice it for a month; then come back to this exploration and see if it becomes easier.

If you feel triggered at the thought of looking out a year into the future, it also could be an indication you are living with trauma or that you are in survival mode. And while those subjects are beyond the scope of this book, this might be an opportunity to bring your circumstances into the light, especially with the help of a trained practitioner. Additionally, somatic practices can be incredibly therapeutic and helpful for releasing old emotions and some of the hidden trauma in our bodies, and you can check out the resources section for ideas on where to start with this.

Sometimes there are things that are truly keeping us stuck in old patterns, and we have to take the courageous first step to start the process of unraveling what's stuck. Other times, it just comes down to making a decision.

You have every right to continue to live in your old belief system, wearing your old brand. But what never changes, never changes. In other words, if things suck now, they're just going to continue to suck, until you make a decision to change. All the power is in your hands. I know you can do it!

30-SECOND SUMMARY

The art of losing weight and keeping it off is *you*. It's what you know, what you believe, and how you see yourself that influence the decisions you make daily.

1. We make the majority of our daily decisions from our subconscious mind. The subconscious mind doesn't rely on willpower to make decisions, so these decisions can occur on autopilot.

2. Most of the time, when we attempt to change a behavior, we go directly to the behavior itself. The problem with this is that we are making decisions about that behavior from our conscious mind and often have to rely on willpower to follow through.

3. In order to see permanent behavior change, we must learn and acquire the skills it takes to shift behavior,

change our beliefs around the behavior, and change our identity as it relates to that behavior.

My hope is that the words and exercises in this chapter strengthened your faith in yourself. Use these exercises over and over again, in every area of your life, when you desire to see change. Once you begin putting the words in this chapter into practice, you will be amazed at how your thoughts—and life—transform.

If fact, you may even find yourself wondering if the changes you quickly see are just beginner's luck, and you may start waiting for the other shoe to drop, on your next vacation or even this upcoming weekend. Don't—that's just an old limiting belief coming up, and I've got your back. In the next chapter, I'll give you clear direction on how to handle everything that life throws at you week after week, so that you never "fall off the wagon" again.

CHAPTER 9

PULLING IT ALL TOGETHER

At this point, my hope is that you are feeling empowered by what you've learned about your body and the power of your mind and how both can help you create an entirely new version of yourself.

So, what is required to apply all this knowledge about your body—and mind—week in and week out?

The first step is the decision to be aware of your choices—intentional and unintentional—from this point forward. And I have an incredibly simple process to help you accomplish that every week.

Yes! Every. Single. Week.

It's a simple three-part process that you can use at home, when you're traveling, or even when you're on vacation. It looks like this:

- **Preview** the week.
- **Live** the week.
- **Review** the week.

This entire process takes about an hour every week, but the amount of time it's going to give back to you—in the short term *and* the long term—is worth every minute.

PREVIEW

The very last thing I do every Friday before picking up my daughter from school is to spend an hour previewing the upcoming week. You can do this on Sunday night or Monday morning—whatever works for you.

1. Empty *everything* swimming around in your head about the upcoming week. *Everything.* Do this by grabbing a pad of paper and jotting down bullet points or typing into the notes app on your phone—whatever works.
    - What is on the calendar for the next week (due dates, happy hours, baseball games, appointments, meetings)?
    - What is not currently on the calendar but needs to be added?
    - What about "housekeeping" stuff like laundry, grocery shopping, or washing the car?
    - How about weekend plans—do you have anything planned or anything you want or need to accomplish?
    - How do the current plans for the week affect breakfast/lunch/dinner?
2. Add the standing meetings you have with your Metabolic Ecosystem. Here are some examples:
    - three strength-training workouts
    - bedtime: lights out by 10:00 p.m. every night
    - 20 minutes of a stress-relieving practice, like breath work or journaling, every day
    - 20-minute brisk walk every day
3. How do the current plans for the week affect mealtimes? What about your nonnegotiables? Will you have to move anything around (such as your kid's baseball game on Wednesday night cutting into meal prep as well as dinner) to accommodate the schedule?
4. Input all of the above into a calendar. I use Google calendar, but any calendar works. This might take a while

the first few times you do it, but once you're used to it, it's
pretty easy.

LIVE

Go about your week, living in alignment with the plan you created in
your preview. The key here is to stick to your calendar as closely as
possible, while understanding that—of course—stuff comes up. Find
some flexibility and let go of the all-or-nothing mentality that the diet
industry taught you. After doing this for a while, you'll wonder how
you ever lived life any other way!

Here's a peek at what my actual week looked like when I was writing this chapter.

Monday

- It's a day packed with meetings, so I made sure to prepare
  meals on the weekend. Using the BYO Meal Guide from
  chapter 2, I added ingredients for smoothies into bags
  and placed them in the freezer so they are ready to mix
  and go. I used frozen blueberries, chia seeds, and cashews,
  and I add protein powder and almond milk as I go. I also
  prepped ground turkey, rice, and broccoli for lunches. I
  already have shredded cheese and avocados on hand and
  could add either as a healthy fat.
- I squeeze in the no-equipment workout from the resources section of the Metabolism Makeover website
  (metabolismmakeover.co) to get my blood flowing between meetings.
- Because I have a screen in my face all day, I am extra diligent to not skip my wind-down activities at night—a hot
  magnesium bath, shower, or sauna session plus reading in
  bed, to help get me into sleep mode.

Tuesday

- Because I have a deadline tomorrow, I know today will be a long day (and night) in front of my laptop, so I plan accordingly with my prepped meals and my favorite healthy takeout for dinner. I order from the steakhouse down the street (a bun-less cheeseburger and fries).
- I take advantage of an appointment for my daughter in the morning and go for a brisk, zone 2 walk while waiting for her.
- I don't get into bed until after midnight, so I take a low dose of melatonin, 200 mg of theanine, and 200 mg of magnesium bisglycinate to help relax my mind and body from the long day.

Wednesday

- The day doesn't start as planned. My daughter wakes me up at 5:45 a.m., so I only get about five hours of sleep. Given this lack of sleep, I skip the strength workout I had planned today and move it to later in the week.
- I also wake up stiff, which often happens after two long workdays in a row, so I incorporate extra movement, mobility work, and stretching into my day.
- I am extra intentional about eating PHFF today, knowing I'll likely have increased cravings and may feel a little hungrier due to the lack of sleep. I eat my planned breakfast and lunch, a protein bar for a snack, and tacos with ground beef, cheese, avocado, lettuce, and tomato on two Siete tortillas for dinner.

Thursday

- I do my rescheduled workout first thing today and get back to work. I always strength train on Wednesday or

Thursday because they are light meeting days and I'm less likely to find a reason to skip.

- Because of the morning workout, I opt for a starchy carb at breakfast instead of my last prepped smoothie. I make sourdough toast with cream cheese, smoked salmon, and avocado and add a scoop of collagen to my coffee.
- I incorporate breaks for breath work throughout the day. No matter how chaotic my schedule gets, I never skip my daily stress-relieving practices. This might be breath work, guided meditation, journaling, acupuncture, or energy work.
- My daughter wants pizza for dinner, so instead of the leftover tacos I had planned, we make a Banza pizza from the freezer and top it with lots of chicken sausage and veggies. We also put together a big salad with broccoli, black olives, cherry tomatoes, and Herby Ranch Dressing. You can find a link to some of my favorite PHFF recipes like this one in the resources section.

Friday

- I do my weekly preview (and review, which we'll get to soon) and set myself up for success the following week.
- I put in a Costco order to come over the weekend; I realize as I'm doing my weekly preview that I'm low on proteins in the house. I get ground beef, chicken thighs (I love doing them in the slow cooker to make shredded chicken), and frozen shrimp, along with frozen blueberries and cherries for smoothies.
- Tonight, the plan is takeout, wine, and a documentary. To make sure I keep my blood sugar as steady as possible while drinking alcohol, I pick a high-protein dinner of grilled shrimp, broccoli, and a large side salad, plus a clean, low-sugar wine like Scout & Cellar to avoid a hangover. I also drink electrolytes in between sips of wine to stay hydrated.

Saturday

- Today, we head to the lake, so I make a big PHFF breakfast, to avoid getting snacky on the boat: breakfast tacos
  with eggs, avocado, spinach, pico de gallo, cilantro, and
  Siete tortillas. We love tacos!
- I also do a strength-training workout in the morning
  because it is a priority to get to the gym on Saturday and
  Sunday to take advantage of the childcare they offer.
- At lunch, I have two vodka sodas and share a plate of nachos with my daughter. I ask for extra chicken on the nachos because the extra protein triggers satiety hormones
  more quickly. (I used to always overeat foods like nachos,
  but now I know how to enjoy them without overdoing it.)
- I have a high-protein, veggie-filled dinner of grilled
  salmon, steak, zucchini, and tomatoes.

Sunday

- Sundays are for lunch dates with my daughter, and we always choose a place that's easy (like Chipotle!) and where
  we can get a good PHFF meal. My usual Chipotle order is
  a chicken or carnitas bowl with white rice (because I like
  it more than brown), cheese, pico de gallo, salsa verde,
  lettuce, and a side of guacamole. My daughter gets a small
  bag of chips with her kids' meal, so we split that with the
  guacamole.
- Like most Sundays, we choose two proteins, one or two
  starchy carbs, and vegetables to cook for the week ahead.
  We sauté shrimp, cook chicken thighs in the slow cooker,
  make rice on the stove, air-fry cauliflower, and zap spaghetti squash in the microwave. As a bonus, we make
  hard-boiled eggs for breakfast and snacks. I also have
  more tortillas on hand, so I know I have lots of options for
  meals next week, such as shrimp scampi with butter and
  spaghetti squash; chicken tacos with avocado; shrimp,

rice, cauliflower, and avocado; or chicken, rice, cauliflower, and avocado.

Now, you might be thinking, *That's great for you, Megan, but if I
ate nachos and drank vodka sodas for lunch, it'd be all downhill from
there.* Or, *If I ate pizza on a Wednesday, I'd experience so much guilt
the rest of the week that it wouldn't even be worth it.*

I get it. It takes practice to overcome the all-or-nothing mentality. But it's completely within your power—and easier than you might
think, especially when you hear Hallie's story.

Most of Hallie's Saturdays started with brunch with her girlfriends. While she was always excited to meet up with her friends for
some downtime, a dark cloud of food anxiety would loom over this
weekly meetup. This was the meal that would sabotage all of Hallie's
hard work during the week and was usually a catalyst for a downward
spiral for the remainder of the weekend. She'd wake up, fast until
brunch, and then order a breakfast burrito, Bloody Mary, a few mimosas, and dessert. After an afternoon nap, Hallie would wake up feeling
bad about herself for having the dessert and sugary mimosas, but even
after all that food, she'd be starving again and would go into "fuck it"
mode and order pizza. This would continue into Sunday, until she'd
wake up on Monday morning feeling bloated, exhausted, and once
again ashamed of her weekend eating.

But once Hallie learned how her body worked and realized her
power and freedom to make a different choice, these brunches started
looking a lot different.

Now, she wakes up on Saturday and makes a smoothie to calm her
hunger, because she knows she isn't really saving calories by getting
hangry and shoveling food down at brunch. She loves her breakfast
burrito and Bloody Mary ritual, so she still orders it. She only eats half
of the burrito, since she's not starving, and decides she'd rather have
another drink instead of getting dessert. The Bloody Mary and burrito
will probably make her a little tired later, and she might have some
carb cravings, too, but she's okay with that. It's worth it. She's already
planning to pick up a bun-less burger for dinner. She leaves brunch
feeling full but satisfied, with no impulse to eat junk food for the rest
of the weekend. She moves on with her day, gets her bun-less burger,

and has another smoothie on Sunday morning. On Monday, Hallie feels happy that she was able to connect with friends over the weekend and is feeling energized and ready to go.

How was Hallie able to make this switch? She used what I like to call the Next Best Choice Framework.

The Next Best Choice Framework

The Next Best Choice Framework is a deliberate process you can use anytime you find yourself in a situation where you are consciously choosing to "stay on track" or "deviate from the track." This might be eating something that won't be blood sugar balancing, staying out later than planned, or skipping a scheduled workout when different plans pop up. When you start to use the Next Best Choice Framework, you'll likely have to consciously walk through each step deliberately. But eventually, this will become a subconscious practice that you won't even have to think about. This right here is your ticket to food freedom. Let's take a look:

1. Pause.
   - When you find yourself in a situation where there is something that you want to eat that isn't necessarily blood sugar balancing or a part of your daily routine, consciously take a beat.
2. Walk through both options.
   - What will happen and how will you feel if you decide to eat this food? How will it be metabolized in your body? How will it make you feel in the moment? In an hour? In four hours? How will you feel emotionally if you eat this food?
   - What will happen and how will you feel if you decide *not* to eat this food? What will you eat instead, if anything? How will you feel in an hour? In four hours? How will you feel emotionally if you decide to skip it?
3. Make a decision, and then make a plan (if needed).
   - If you decide *not* to eat the food, cool.

- If you decide to eat the food, that's also okay! Just ask yourself, *What is the next best choice that I can make after eating this food?* This might be choosing what other foods to eat *with* the food you chose, or it might be planning how you'll handle a potential blood sugar crash later.

The Next Best Choice Framework works beautifully in situations where you're able to start with the first step—pause.

But sometimes humans don't pause. Sometimes we bulldoze. Sometimes we have one too many glasses of vino, and the pause button is no longer accessible. Sometimes a bag of Tostitos and a bowl of queso are set in front of us, and we black out until it's gone. And guess what? This *will* happen. It's not a matter of *if*, it's when. So then what?

You still get to use the framework! It just looks a little different:

1. Pause.
   - When you find yourself in a situation where you've gone off the rails, take a beat, come back to the present moment, and remind yourself that *you did not fail, because you cannot fail at this.*
2. Walk through what happens next.
   - How will this food be metabolized in your body? Was it carbohydrate/sugar heavy? Are you going to experience a blood sugar crash later? If so, what can you do next? What can you do to feel better in the moment?
3. Make a plan.
   - Decide what happens next. Go for a walk to stabilize blood sugar or get in a resistance workout so that your muscle glycogen can soak up some of those wonderful carbs for strength building. Decide on your next blood-sugar-balancing meal. Drink water. Breathe.

While you're practicing the Next Best Choice Framework, remember that the right answer is whatever solution you come up with—full stop. This is the antiperfectionism framework that you've been missing in every diet you've done in the past.

As you might remember, the pillar that I struggle with most is sleep, which is why I have to be very diligent about my bedtime and evening wind-down routine. Sometimes, though, I find myself having to use the Next Best Choice Framework when it comes to logging my zzz's. Here's an example:

1. Pause.
   - I'm faced with the decision to spend quality time with my partner in the evening or to get eight hours of sleep.
2. Walk through both options.
   - Because of our schedules, if I forego time with my partner now, I will miss that connection with him this week. We have some things we need to talk about, and missing our date night could result in pushing issues under the rug, which will likely cause more chronic stress than getting less than eight hours of sleep for one night.
   - Though if I decide to go through with date night, I'll have some sleep debt, which may cause me to not be totally on point tomorrow at work, and it'll likely cause my hunger cues to be off.
3. Make a decision, and then make a plan (if needed).
   - I choose date night. I'll push my 8:00 a.m. meeting to 10:00 a.m. (if possible), when I know I'll be more alert. I've got my smoothie planned for breakfast, my lunch prepped, and a high-protein snack that should keep me satisfied throughout the workday. I'll push my work-out to the day after so that my body can be adequately recovered from a night of less sleep.

Being intentional about our choices takes us off autopilot and into the present moment. We're able to make decisions about our bodies and our lives that will serve our highest good—even if that decision isn't the "best" decision for our immediate health. Would your body prefer that you skip the donut? Sure. Would it prefer that you get eight hours of sleep? Definitely. But we are human beings performing a daily circus act called life, and sometimes the donut date with your daughter or date night with your partner is worth it.

When you can stay present, instead of spiraling out of control, you can take the time to reflect and say, *I ate two bowls of pasta because I skipped my afternoon snack and got too hungry.* That mental note can carry over so that you make a point to prioritize your afternoon snack.

Diet Danger Zones

Sound the alarm—we're about to enter the Diet Danger Zones.

You know what I'm talking about. Those scenarios that your latest "diet" didn't prepare you for or when it advises you to just order the salad. Of course, that doesn't work because either you're not going to order the salad *or* you're going to follow up the salad with two martinis and a milkshake to satisfy yourself.

I'm talking about vacations, holidays, happy hours, travel, and, well, even weekends. These infamous Diet Danger Zones pull you off track quickly and often result in having to "start over."

Lucky for you, Diet Danger Zones no longer have to exist in your world because these situations are just *life* when you feel in control and know how to handle them. You can—and should!—use the Next Best Choice Framework in these situations, but here are some additional tools to help set you up mentally and biologically for success:

1. **Create a minimal morning routine:** What can you do every day that will help you set your tone for the day? It could be something as simple as drinking a glass of water, walking for 10 minutes while returning emails, and then making a smoothie. This communicates to your brain that vacation, weekends, and high-stress mornings are the same as a regular Tuesday. You'll be far more likely to treat your body like you would on a regular Tuesday if you start your day like one.

2. **Pack 911 "mini-meals":** This is a great weekend travel hack. Instead of relying on the cooler of snacks, pack mini-meals so that you're not chowing down on gummy

worms every 30 minutes. Some good options are hard-boiled eggs with veggies and dip, turkey and cheese with grapes, or whole-food protein bars.

3. **Pick one meal for indulging:** This is a go-to vacation tip. It's as simple as it sounds—when you're on a trip, pick one indulgent meal each day and eat PHFF for the rest. For example, breakfast might be a quick protein coffee at the Airbnb, lunch could be some steak taco lettuce wraps with guacamole, and then at dinner, go nuts.

4. **Choose one starchy carb:** This is my favorite tip for going out to eat. If you really want a burger and fries, decide if you'd prefer the fries or the bun on the burger. Do a bun-less burger and fries or a regular burger with a veggie side.

5. **Protein and healthy fat first:** I love this tip for parties, barbecues, and holidays. Fill your plate with PHFF first. This could be shrimp cocktail, vegetables, guacamole, hot wings, nuts, and bites from the meat-and-cheese tray. At a cookout, this could be a cheeseburger (no bun), coleslaw, grilled veggies, and some deviled eggs you brought along to share. Then pick one or two starchy carbs that you love, have a serving, and move on. If you're not immediately filling up on snacky things like chips, bread, and brownies, you'll be far less likely to overindulge.

6. **Alcohol and sugar don't mix:** Sugar is public enemy number one when you are consuming alcohol. It can cause massive blood sugar swings, and the body will prioritize clearing alcohol from your system over your metabolism any day. Skip sweetened mixers, sugary wines, liqueurs, and high-carb beers. No-sugar mixers with hard liquor and clean, low-sugar wines are your best bet. If you're out and about, remember that it's okay to make substitutions when ordering a drink. Skip the simple syrup and honey. Ask for club soda instead of tonic or Sprite. Order a margarita with tequila, a little orange liqueur, fresh lime, and no agave.

7. **Sober on weeknights:** As an alternative to "dry January," every New Year I challenge my clients to save alcohol for weekends only. It's a way to sustainably reduce alcohol intake without the all-or-nothing mentality that often backfires come February. This works best with an accountability partner, so grab a friend!

8. **Hack your hangover:** The handful of vodka sodas you drink on a Saturday night is not causing weight gain. The hangover-causing binge fest is. Instead of lying around ordering takeout all day, have PHFF-friendly versions of your favorite hangover foods ready to go.

Remember the beginning of the book when I said I'm going to teach you how to take back your power over food? This is it.

You now have the tools you need to navigate even the most challenging situations and feel confident in making the right choices for your body day by day and moment by moment. Whether you're at the beach, nursing a breakup, or having girlfriends over for "wine-down Wednesday."

So far, you've previewed, planned, and lived your week, and it's once again time to preview your upcoming week. But first, you're going to take just a few minutes to complete one critical step before the next week begins.

REVIEW

Before doing your weekly preview, take a few minutes to review the previous week.

Doing an end-of-week review is not a concept I came up with—it's a classic productivity hack for those of us who consistently use phrases like "I don't have time" and "life is too chaotic right now."

The process of this review is far less important than the intention behind it, which is pulling yourself out of autopilot. It's giving you the opportunity to live your life with intention. It's a chance to get honest with yourself and build self-awareness. It's a way to look at what went well and what didn't and then to create positive change next week by using that information.

If you make this review a priority in your life, you will never look back and think, *WTF was I doing all these years, and where did the time go?*

This practice takes only 5–10 minutes but can create so much space in your week, while still prioritizing yourself. I do this by asking myself the following questions and journaling about them, but you can do whatever works best for you:

- Was I well prepared with PHFF options all week?
- Did I fit in my goal number of strength-training sessions?
- Did I move as much as I intended to?
- Did I get an adequate amount of sleep for my body?
- Did I make time to incorporate stress-relieving activities?
- Did I take care of my gut by eating a variety of fibrous and fermented foods?

Here's what my review would look like after the week I outlined at the beginning of the chapter:

I was prepared with PHFF options all week and was really intentional, using the Next Best Choice, if I deviated. I got four strength workouts in, but I didn't move as much as I had intended. Next week, I'll schedule my walks during calls or during other times I can better habit stack. I didn't get nearly enough sleep on Tuesday night, and if I had to do it again, I would have NOT chosen to stay up late. It's never worth how I feel the next day. Next time, I'll choose waking up early over staying up late. I did really well making time for stress-relieving practices and I ate a wide variety of fibrous foods, but I do need to add raw pickles and plain Greek yogurt to my grocery list for next week to up my fermented foods consumption.

And now I can move right into my weekly preview and start implementing these new strategies.

This is it, friends. You now have the tools you need to make over your metabolism! But how will you know if it's working? Let's next set some expectations as you get started.

THE TRUE MEASURE OF PROGRESS

Don't forget—the diet industry has conditioned you to believe that long-term results are available to you instantaneously.

So this is a good spot to pause and remind you that:

Sustainable weight loss *should* take time.

Sustainable weight loss *should* take time.

Sustainable weight loss *should* take time.

Some of you will see inches gone within the first 30 days, some of you will see slow and steady progress over months, and others won't see the scale budge until they're consistent for three or four months. For others, it may take even longer and may require additional lab work to see what other issues might be at play. Regardless of which camp you fall into, it's time to remove any pressure you are putting on yourself to have a brand-new body by next month.

If it's not abundantly clear by now, I'm not interested in rapid weight loss, quick-fix results, or shredded abs that you kill yourself to manufacture. And I'm sure Alex from chapter 1 would back me up on this after she gained all her weight back and felt miserable in the process.

Instead, I'm interested in making sure you feel confident and proud in your skin for many years to come. I care about you being so in tune with your body that you know exactly what it's asking for every moment of every day.

I want you to have so much trust in yourself that you don't listen to a damn word from anyone about what you should or shouldn't be doing to your precious temple. And that includes me!

Of course, I recommend using the guidelines in this book to get started. But once you begin feeling more and more in tune with your body—and you will—listen to your intuition and feed your body what it needs. More carbs? Less carbs? More protein at breakfast? It's not witchcraft. It's just body awareness. Now you have it, and you'll continue to fine-tune it over time. This is so exciting!

PAST DIETER PROFILE

Joe thought I was crazy when I told him that his body would start telling him what it needed. He laughed and said the only thing his body tells him he needs is Budweiser. After just two weeks of eating PHFF, Joe was out to eat (okay, he was having a few beers) with friends and found himself thinking he needed to eat some protein, so he ordered a bun-less burger. He couldn't believe it!

As a reminder from chapter 3, there is absolutely no reason to use a scale, unless you care about a number on the scale more than you care about how you look and feel in your body *and* that number on the scale has zero effect on your mental or physical health. I'm guessing that's about 1 percent of you reading this—tops. In the end, those numbers don't mean anything beyond the meaning that you assign to them.

Head back to chapter 3 to refresh your memory on using measurements or mirror selfies to track your progress. I can't tell you how many times I've had this exact conversation:

Client: "I'm so frustrated the scale hasn't budged."

Me: "What about measurements? Have you been tracking those as well?"

Client: "Oh, yes! I've lost several inches, and I can definitely tell by looking in the mirror. But I just can't figure out why the scale won't move, and I'm getting really discouraged."

Me: "Put the scale in the trash, please."

Once you begin to put some muscle on your body, the scale may stay the same as you see your pants size drop. This is great! It means you are adding fat-burning, anti-inflammatory muscle and burning inflammatory fat.

Every year, I run a "toss the scale" challenge for my clients for an entire month. The purpose of this challenge is to observe what happens throughout the day when you don't weigh yourself in the morning. How do you approach food differently? Do you tune into your hunger and satiety hormones more if you're not thinking about what the scale said? What's your overall mood like, compared with when you step on the scale every morning? If you're really addicted to the scale, and you think it's affecting your mood or the way you eat, I challenge you to toss the scale for a month!

PAST DIETER PROFILE

Diana had been stuck in a plateau for months. She knew she wasn't perfect, but she still felt like she was doing all the right things, even if she wasn't totally consistent—eating PHFF, exercising, sleeping well, and managing her stress. After just one month of ditching the scale, Diana lost three inches, her pants fit better, and she felt more energized! She realized the scale had been dictating her mood—and her food choices. Even though she was still indulging from time to time, she found herself much more intentional about it and never again had to deal with a "bad scale day."

YOU'RE DOING IT!

Don't underestimate the shifts you've already made while reading this book. Even if you haven't yet implemented a single thing you've learned, you're already experiencing a new sense of freedom. You're already becoming the next version of you.

It doesn't matter if you have to use the Next Best Choice Framework to get back on track for the next 100 days in a row. *What matters is that you love yourself enough to keep going.*

Your curiosity about your body and your willingness to do the difficult, vulnerable work in chapter 8 tells me that you are already becoming the next version of yourself that you dreamed up when completing that exercise. All the shifts you're feeling—even if they are still so small—will add up over time. One day, you'll wake up and say, *Wait, did I really do this? Is this the new me?*

My hope in writing this book is to show you that there is a life on the other side of obsessing over food and your weight. Because you were willing to take that leap of faith and go on this journey with me, that life is already available to you; in fact, you're already living it!

As I finish up this chapter almost exactly one year after typing the first words of the initial draft, I am feeling overwhelmed by pride for your commitment to yourself and your willingness to push yourself to try something different. It probably seems weird that I could care so much about someone I don't know (and, at this very moment, hasn't even read this book yet), but just like Alex from chapter 1, *I was a version of you* at one time. I have been where you are, felt everything that you're feeling, and thought everything that you're thinking.

And that's how I know that, just like me, you'll move forward with imperfect progress from here on out. Because this is it—there is no continuity program. You'll go in and out of different seasons of life, and you'll be equipped to handle each and every one of them. Your metabolism makeover—and new life—starts now.

ACKNOWLEDGMENTS

Big shout-out to my team of human angels, especially Cierra Robbins and Helena Hansen, who supported me, put up with me, and gave me the space to be creative during the writing process. I owe a huge thanks to my entire Metabolism Makeover community: YOU brought this book to life with me. Another big thanks to Elizabeth Marshall, who pulled this message out of me, guided me through the process of self-publishing, and was my emotional support partner from start to finish. Thanks to the Girl Friday Productions team for believing in this book and my mission and, in particular, Audra Figgins, because editors are superheroes. Les McGowen—wow!—thank you for pushing me to write this book. Thank you to my personal development team, healers, and friends Lyndsey Chambers, Kelly Gamble, Sheila Polstein, and Sarah Elkany. Thank you, Megan Anderson, for putting T. to bed and holding my life together for many months while I finished this book. Mom and Dad, thank you for being excited for me with each new venture and never once trying to hold me back to keep me safe. Finally, S., you are my mirror. Thank you for continually pulling me out of my own way.

REFERENCES

In this section, I've put together some of the most important and relevant studies, articles, and experts that support what you've learned in this book. I've organized them by topic for easy reference.

DIETING/WEIGHT LOSS

Centers for Disease Control and Prevention (June 3, 2022) "About adult BMI." Centers for Disease Control and Prevention. Accessed November 8, 2022. https://www.cdc.gov/healthyweight/assessing/bmi/adult_bmi/index.html.

Davy, S. R., Benes, B. A., and Driskell, J. A. (2006) "Sex differences in dieting trends, eating habits, and nutrition beliefs of a group of midwestern college students." *Journal of the Academy of Nutrition and Dietetics* 106 (10): 1673–77. https://doi.org/10.1016/j.jada.2006.07.017.

Marketdata (2022) *The U.S. weight loss market: 2022 status report & forecast.* Accessed November 9, 2022. https://www.researchandmarkets.com/r/31b44w.

Popkin, B. M., and Hawkes, C. (2016) "Sweetening of the global diet, particularly beverages: Patterns, trends, and policy responses." *Lancet: Diabetes & Endocrinology* 4 (2): 174–86. https://doi.org/10.1016/s2213-8587(15)00419-2.

Rolls, B. J., Fedoroff, I. C., and Guthrie, J. F. (1991) "Gender differences in eating behavior and body weight regulation." *Health Psychology*

10 (2): 133–42. https://doi.org/10.1037/0278-6133.10.2.133.

San-Millán, I., and Brooks, G. A. (2018) "Assessment of metabolic flexibility by means of measuring blood lactate, fat, and carbohydrate oxidation responses to exercise in professional endurance athletes and less-fit individuals." *Sports Medicine* 48: 467–79. https://doi.org/10.1007/s40279-017-0751-x.

MACRONUTRIENTS

DiNicolantonio, J., and O'Keefe, J. H. (2021) "Does fish oil reduce the risk of cardiovascular events and death? Recent level 1 evidence says yes: Pro: Fish oil is useful to prevent or treat cardiovascular disease." *Missouri Medicine* 118 (3): 214–218. Accessed November 14, 2022. https://pubmed.ncbi.nlm.nih.gov/34149080.

Di Stefano, S. (June 23, 2016) "The myth of optimal protein intake." Mind Pump Media. Accessed November 14, 2022. https://www.mindpumpmedia.com/blog/the-myth-of-optimal-protein-intake.

Harris, W. S., Mozaffarian, D., Lefevre, M., Toner, C. D., Colombo, J., Cunnane, S. C., Holden, J. M., et al. (2009) "Towards establishing dietary reference intakes for eicosapentaenoic and docosahexaenoic acids." *Journal of Nutrition* 139 (4): 804S–19S. https://doi.org/10.3945/jn.108.101329.

Hu, F. B., Stampfer, M. J., Manson, J. E., Rimm, E., Colditz, G. A., Rosner, B. A., Hennekens, C. H., et al. (1997) "Dietary fat intake and the risk of coronary heart disease in women." *New England Journal of Medicine* 337: 1491–99. https://doi.org/10.1056/nejm199711203372102.

Institute of Medicine (2005) *Dietary reference intakes for energy, carbohydrate, fiber, fat, fatty acids, cholesterol, protein, and amino acids.* Washington, DC: National Academies Press. https://doi.org/10.17226/10490.

Lyon, G. (May 23, 2020) "Are you committing carb-o-cide?" YouTube. Accessed November 8, 2022. https://www.youtube.com/watch?v=Cg1Ng4JwxpA.

Martínez-González, M. Á., and Sánchez-Villegas, A. (2004) "Review:

The emerging role of Mediterranean diets in cardiovascular epidemiology: Monounsaturated fats, olive oil, red wine or the whole pattern." *European Journal of Epidemiology* 19 (1): 9–13. https://doi.org/10.1023/b:ejep.0000013351.60227.7b.

Mensink, R. P., Zock, P. L., Kester, A. D. M., and Katan, M. B. (2003) "Effects of dietary fatty acids and carbohydrates on the ratio of serum total to HDL cholesterol and on serum lipids and apolipoproteins: A meta-analysis of 60 controlled trials." *American Journal of Clinical Nutrition* 77 (5): 1146–55. https://doi.org/10.1093/ajcn/77.5.1146.

Patterson, E., Wall, R., Fitzgerald, G. F., Ross, R. P., and Stanton, C. (2012) "Health implications of high dietary omega-6 polyunsaturated fatty acids." *Journal of Nutrition and Metabolism* 2012: 1–16. https://doi.org/10.1155/2012/539426.

Phillips, S. M., and Van Loon, L. J. C. (2011) "Dietary protein for athletes: From requirements to optimum adaptation." *Journal of Sports Sciences* 29 (Suppl. 1): S29–S38. https://doi.org/10.1080/02640414.2011.619204.

Power, E., and Rupsis, L. (hosts) (November 17, 2021) "Dr. Gabrielle Lyon: We aren't over fat, we are under muscled." Episode in: *Health Coach Radio* (podcast). Accessed November 8, 2022. https://podcasts.apple.com/au/podcast/we-arent-over-fat-we-are-under-muscled-dr-gabrielle-lyon/id1453608008?i=1000542247128.

STRENGTH AND MOVEMENT

Attia, P. (host) (December 23, 2019) "Iñigo San Millán, Ph.d.: Zone 2 training and metabolic health." Episode 85 in: *The Peter Attia Drive* (podcast). Accessed May 19, 2022. https://peterattiamd.com/inigosanmillan.

Bowman, K. (February 1, 2016) "What is nutritious movement?" YouTube. Accessed December 15, 2022. https://www.youtube.com/watch?v=eeN8efGa6C0.

Buckley, J. P., Mellor, D. D., Morris, M., and Joseph, F. (2013)

"Standing-based office work shows encouraging signs of attenuating post-prandial glycaemic excursion." *Occupational and Environmental Medicine* 71 (2): 109–11. https://doi.org/10.1136/oemed-2013-101823.

Colberg, S. R., Zarrabi, L., Bennington, L., Nakave, A., Thomas Somma, C., Swain, D. P., and Sechrist, S. R. (2009) "Postprandial walking is better for lowering the glycemic effect of dinner than pre-dinner exercise in type 2 diabetic individuals." *Journal of Post-acute and Long-term Care Medicine* 10 (6): 394–97. https://doi.org/10.1016/j.jamda.2009.03.015.

Erickson, M. L., Jenkins, N. T., and McCully, K. K. (2017) "Exercise after you eat: Hitting the postprandial glucose target." *Frontiers in Endocrinology* 8. https://doi.org/10.3389/fendo.2017.00228.

Huberman, A. (host) (August 15, 2022) "Dr. Peter Attia: Exercise, nutrition, hormones for vitality & longevity." Episode in: *Huberman Lab* (podcast). Scicomm Media. Accessed August 17, 2022. https://podcasts.apple.com/us/podcast/dr-peter-attia-exercise-nutrition-hormones-for-vitality/id1545953110?i=1000576100900.

Paluch, A. E., Bajpai, S., Bassett, D. R., Carnethon, M. R., Ekelund, U., Evenson, K. R., Galuska, D. A., et al. (2022) "Daily steps and all-cause mortality: A meta-analysis of 15 international cohorts." *Lancet Public Health* 7 (3): E219–28. https://doi.org/10.1016/s2468-2667(21)00302-9.

BETTER SLEEP

Academy of General Dentistry (April 6, 2010) "Mouth breathing can cause major health problems." Science Daily. Accessed November 6, 2022. https://www.sciencedaily.com/releases/2010/04/100406125714.htm.

Al Khatib, H. K., Harding, S. V., Darzi, J., and Pot, G. K. (2016) "The effects of partial sleep deprivation on energy balance: A systematic review and meta-analysis." *European Journal of Clinical Nutrition* 71 (5): 614–24. https://doi.org/10.1038/ejcn.2016.201.

Centers for Disease Control and Prevention (February 18, 2016) "1 in 3 adults don't get enough sleep." Centers for Disease Control and

Prevention. Accessed November 8, 2022. https://www.cdc.gov /media/releases/2016/p0215-enough-sleep.html.

Greenfield, B. (host) (September 19, 2015) "The man behind the advanced sleep hacking tactics used by the world's most elite athletes: Meet Nick Littlehales." Episode in: *Ben Greenfield Life* (podcast). Accessed August 19, 2022. https://bengreenfieldlife.com /podcast/sleep-podcasts/sleep-hacking-tactics-with-nick -littlehales.

Hanlon, E. C., Tasali, E., Leproult, R., Stuhr, K. L., Doncheck, E., de Wit, H., Hillard, C. J., et al. (2016) "Sleep restriction enhances the daily rhythm of circulating levels of endocannabinoid 2-arachidonoylglycerol." *Sleep* 39 (3): 653–64. https://doi .org/10.5665/sleep.5546.

Johns Hopkins Medicine (August 8, 2021) "The science of sleep: Understanding what happens when you sleep." Johns Hopkins Medicine. Accessed November 8, 2022. https://www.hopkins medicine.org/health/wellness-and-prevention/the-science-of -sleep-understanding-what-happens-when-you-sleep.

Nedeltcheva, A. V., Kilkus, J. M., Imperial, J., Schoeller, D. A., and Penev, P. D. (2010) "Insufficient sleep undermines dietary efforts to reduce adiposity." *Annals of Internal Medicine* 153 (7): 435–41. https://doi.org/10.7326/0003-4819-153-7-201010050-00006.

Schwab, R. J. (2022) "Snoring." In: "Neurologic disorders: Sleep and wakefulness disorders." Merck Manual, Professional Version. Accessed November 8, 2022. https://www.merckmanuals.com /professional/neurologic-disorders/sleep-and-wakefulness -disorders/snoring.

Taheri, S., Lin, L., Austin, D., Young, T., and Mignot, E. (2004) "Short sleep duration is associated with reduced leptin, elevated ghrelin, and increased body mass index." *PLoS Medicine* 1 (3): e62. https://doi.org/10.1371/journal.pmed.0010062.

Tasali, E., Wroblewski, K., Kahn, E., Kilkus, J., and Schoeller, D. A. (2022) "Effect of sleep extension on objectively assessed energy intake among adults with overweight in real-life settings." *JAMA Internal Medicine* 182 (4): 365–74. https://doi.org/10.1001 /jamainternmed.2021.8098.

Walker, M. (n.d.) "Matthew Walker teaches the science of better sleep" (online class). MasterClass. Accessed November 8, 2022. https://www.masterclass.com/classes/matthew-walker-teaches -the-science-of-better-sleep.

Watson, N. F., Badr, M. S., Belenky, G., Bliwise, D. L., Buxton, O. M., Buysse, D., Dinges, D. F., et al. (2015) "Recommended amount of sleep for a healthy adult: A joint consensus statement of the American Academy of Sleep Medicine and Sleep Research Society." *Sleep* 38 (6): 843–44. https://doi.org/10.5665/sleep.4716.

STRESS MANAGEMENT

American Psychological Association (n.d.) "Stress in America." American Psychological Association. Accessed November 8, 2022. https://www.apa.org/news/press/releases/stress.

Castillo, B. (January 19, 2022) "What is the Get Coached Model?" The Life Coach School. Accessed November 8, 2022. https://thelife coachschool.com/self-coaching-model-guide.

Edwards, M. K., and Loprinzi, P. D. (2018) "Experimental effects of brief, single bouts of walking and meditation on mood profile in young adults." *Health Promotion Perspectives* 8 (3): 171–78. https://www.ncbi.nlm.nih.gov/pmc/articles/PMC6064756.

Goldstein, M. R., Lewin, R. K., and Allen, J. J. (2020) "Improvements in well-being and cardiac metrics of stress following a yogic breathing workshop: Randomized controlled trial with active comparison." *Journal of American College Health* 70 (3): 918–28. https://doi.org/10.1080/07448481.2020.1781867.

Monat, A., and Lazarus, R. S. (editors) (1991) *Stress and Coping: An Anthology.* 3rd ed. New York: Columbia University Press.

North Dakota State University (2011) "Walking can help relieve stress." Extension and Ag Research News. Accessed November 8, 2022. https://www.ag.ndsu.edu/news/newsreleases/2011 /aug-8-2011/walking-can-help-relieve-stress.

Pahwa, R., Goyal, A., and Jialal, I. (2022) *Chronic inflammation* (internet). Treasure Island, Fla.: StatPearls Publishing. Updated August 8, 2022. Accessed August 17, 2022. https://www.ncbi.nlm.nih.gov /books/NBK493173.

Tan, S. Y., and Yip, A. (2018) "Hans Selye (1907–1982): Founder of the stress theory." *Singapore Medical Journal* 59 (4): 170–71. https://doi.org/10.11622/smedj.2018043.

A HEALTHY GUT

Huberman, A. (host) (March 7, 2022) "Dr. Justin Sonnenburg: How to build, maintain & repair gut health." Episode in: *Huberman Lab* (podcast). Scicomm Media. Accessed June 7, 2022. https://podcasts.apple.com/us/podcast/dr-justin-sonnenburg-how-to-build-maintain-repair-gut/id1545953110?i=1000553144505.

Pollan, M. (2009) *In defense of food: An eater's manifesto.* New York: Penguin.

Terry, N., and Margolis, K. G. (2016) "Serotonergic mechanisms regulating the GI tract: Experimental evidence and therapeutic relevance." In: Greenwood–Van Meerveld, B. (editor) *Gastrointestinal Pharmacology*. Edinburgh: Springer, Cham, 319–42. https://doi.org/10.1007/164_2016_103.

Wastyk, H. C., Fragiadakis, G. K., Perelman, D., Dahan, D., Merrill, B. D., Yu, F. B., Topf, M., et al. (2021) "Gut-microbiota-targeted diets modulate human immune status." *Cell* 184 (16): 4137–4153. e14. https://doi.org/10.1016/j.cell.2021.06.019.

MINDSET

Darley, J. M., and Batson, C. D. (1973) "'From Jerusalem to Jericho': A study of situational and dispositional variables in helping behavior." *Journal of Personality and Social Psychology* 27 (1): 100–108. https://doi.org/10.1037/h0034449.

Hardy, B. (December 21, 2021) "This 10-minute routine will increase your clarity and creativity." Medium. Accessed November 14, 2022. https://medium.com/@benjaminhardy/this-10-minute-routine-will-increase-your-clarity-and-creativity-94d3ad0249a7.

Morsella, E., Godwin, C. A., Jantz, T. K., Krieger, S., and Gazzaley, A. (2016) "Homing in on consciousness in the nervous system: An

action-based synthesis." *Behavioral and Brain Sciences* 39: E168.
doi:10.1017/S0140525X15000643.

Oakwater, H. (May 29, 2018) "Robert Dilts explains NLP Logical
Levels of learning & change + impact of trauma (part 1)."
YouTube. Accessed November 8, 2022. https://www.youtube.com
/watch?v=hrK9_ZPo790.

RESOURCES

There is only so much you can squeeze into one book, so this section serves as an extension of resources for you, to make life easier as you begin to incorporate what you've learned in the previous chapters. I've compiled a short list of good places to get information, products, and other resources to help you along the way. This list is constantly growing and evolving, so if you'd like more up-to-date suggestions, please go to the Metabolism Makeover website (metabolismmakeover.co /resources), and I will keep you in the loop.

PHFF ESSENTIALS: WHAT'S ALWAYS IN MY KITCHEN

Here is a peek inside my kitchen! I follow the BYO Meal Guide more than I make actual recipes, because I find it to be quicker and easier for meal prep. I actually looked inside my freezer, refrigerator, and pantry to create this list; my staples remain pretty steady, and I wanted to give you some of my favorite, "Megan-approved" brands to look for. Typically, I'll make a couple of proteins, vegetables, and starchy carbs at the beginning of the week and combine them as I go, adding fat to each meal.

Proteins

I love stopping at Costco for organic (or not!) proteins. Buy these in bulk to save lots of cash!

- beef sticks (CHOMPS)
- organic chicken breasts, chicken thighs, ground beef, and wild shrimp (Costco)
- organic deli turkey (Costco)
- eggs from pastured chickens (from local farm CSA)
- protein/collagen powders: Drink Wholesome Meal Replacement Powder, Kion Whey Protein, Truvani Plant-Based Protein, and Collagen Peptides (Further Food or Perfect Supplements)
- protein bars: Nash Bar, RXBAR, and Paleovalley

Healthy Fats

- avocados
- cashews, pistachios, and Brazil nuts (Thrive Market)
- cashew butter (Georgia Grinders)
- cheese (I mix it up, but Kerrygold cheddar and fresh mozzarella are favorites)
- coconut milk (Thrive Market)
- guacamole cups (Costco)
- hummus cups (Costco)
- olives
- pesto (Gotham Greens)

Fiber

- chia seeds (Thrive Market)
- frozen organic berries (Costco)
- frozen organic vegetables (Costco)
- microgreens
- prepped raw or cooked vegetables like broccoli, cauliflower, cucumbers, and carrots
- salad greens

Starchy Carbs

- avocado-oil potato chips (Siete or Thrive Market)
- beans (any kind)
- crackers (Simple Mills)
- grain-free tortilla chips (Siete or Thrive Market)
- jasmine rice (Lundberg)
- potatoes (we do a variety!)
- pasta (Banza, Jovial, and Tolerant Foods)

Condiments/Sauces

- marinara (Rao's)
- bone broth (Kettle & Fire)
- coconut aminos (Bragg)
- mustard, Dijon and yellow
- salsa (any kind without added sugar)
- vinegar: apple cider, balsamic, red, and rice wine (Thrive Market)
- mineral salts (Redmond Real Salt)

Treats

- dark chocolate (Hu and Thrive Market)
- full-fat ice cream (Alden's)

Alcohol

I'm not much of a drinker anymore, but if I do drink, this is what I pick up.

- Dry Farm Wines
- Scout & Cellar
- unflavored vodka, gin, tequila, rum, or whiskey with no

added sugar (Thrive Market)
- club soda, mineral water, or seltzer
- fresh fruit, cucumber slices, and herbs for garnish
- lemons and limes

PHFF RECIPES

Find my favorite PHFF recipes at metabolismmakeover.co/resources.

WORKOUTS

In chapter 3, you found a one-month strength-training program, and at metabolismmakeover.co/resources, you will find the videos that go along with this program, plus a no-equipment program for beginners, travel, or those days you just need to squeeze something in on your living room floor. If you're taking on the one-month program, you will need

- two or three sets of dumbbells or resistance bands (keep in mind, as you progress, you'll need to gradually go up in weight);
- a bench.

There is no need to buy fancy equipment. You can often find dumbbells at consignment stores or secondhand online for a great price. Fabric dumbbells (rather than metal) tend to be the most comfortable to hold. As for a bench, you may be able to find something around the house, like an ottoman or decorative bench (just make sure it's sturdy!).

SLEEP TOOLS

There are so many cool sleep tools on the market, but many of them can be pricey. My advice is to start small, and once you've done the foundational free stuff (morning light! less blue light in the evening!) and you begin to see improvements, add another tool or two to optimize. The following are two relatively inexpensive sleep tools that I use and recommend most often.

Rise App (risescience.com)

This app helps track your sleep debt, and it is wonderful for holding you accountable on sleep. You'll notice that as sleep debt increases, energy decreases. I personally work hard to keep sleep debt under 10 hours (in a two-week cycle), because I know that once I hit 10 hours, my energy levels really tank.

Bon Charge Blue-Light Blockers (boncharge.com)

There are plenty of blue-light blockers on the market, but I like these because they are high-quality *and* stylish. Make sure your blue-light blockers have been tested for effectiveness and that they are a red tint (which is what blocks out blue light at night).

GUT RESOURCES

You'll find the recommended supplements from chapter 7 in the "Supplement Brands" section. Here are a few of the well-researched, easy-to-read books that I've found particularly helpful in the gut-health space:

- *Fiber Fueled: The Plant-Based Gut Health Program for Losing Weight, Restoring Your Health, and Optimizing Your Microbiome* by Will Bulsiewicz
- *The Good Gut: Taking Control of Your Weight, Your Mood, and Your Long-Term Health* by Justin Sonnenburg and Erica Sonnenburg
- *The Mind-Gut Connection: How the Hidden Conversation*

Within Our Bodies Impacts Our Mood, Our Choices, and Our Overall Health by Emeran Mayer

HEALING RESOURCES

Here I've included a few resources from both chapter 6 and chapter 8 as starting points for you.

Emotional Freedom Technique (EFT)/tapping: This is a practice that uses tapping with your fingertips on specific points of the body while talking through traumatic memories and emotions. Tapping sends signals directly to the amygdala, the stress center in the brain. See more at the Tapping Solution Foundation (tappingsolutionfoundation .org).

Inner-child work: This can be particularly helpful to do with a trained therapist, but you absolutely can do inner-child work on your own too. The inner child is a metaphorical "little you"—the part of you who is still childlike and innocent. It can give you a lot of insight into why you repeat dysfunctional patterns and self-sabotaging behavior. Find out more at Rising Woman (risingwoman.com/inner -child-work-healing-trauma-self-acceptance).

Somatic therapy: Somatic therapy theory states that sensations from past trauma may become trapped in the body. There are a number of ways to release this trauma from the body. I've included two resources as places to start:

- *The Body Keeps the Score: Brain, Mind, and Body in the Healing of Trauma* by Bessel van der Kolk
- Ergos Institute of Somatic Education (somaticexperiencing.com)

Breath work: SOMA Breath (somabreath.com) and the Wim Hof Method (wimhofmethod.com).

SUPPLEMENT BRANDS

Targeted supplementation can be a game changer for many, but the supplement industry is the Wild West; choosing pure, high-quality supplements is necessary, unless you want to flush your money down the toilet (literally—if you're taking supplements your body can't even absorb, you'll be flushing them down the toilet). Here are some of my absolute favorite, trusted brands.

Jigsaw: I especially love their electrolytes and magnesium products, but I would recommend any of their supplements.

Just Thrive: One of the only probiotics clinically proven to "arrive alive" in the gut, where it belongs.

LMNT: If you're doing sweaty workouts, saunas, coffee enemas, or anything that is particularly dehydrating, LMNT is a high-sodium electrolyte product that will help replace what you lose through sweat.

Paleovalley: I love their convenient bone-broth powder, grass-fed-beef sticks, and apple-cinnamon bars for a high-protein snack.

Perfect Supplements: My favorite brand for collagen powder, gelatin, whole-food vitamin C, desiccated liver, and a multiorgan product.

Rayvi: A potassium-rich mineral drink made with organic, whole-food ingredients

Re-Lyte: Another tasty electrolyte powder with bioavailable vitamins and minerals.

Urban Moonshine Digestive Bitters: This is the brand of bitters I use, but there are many good brands out there. I prefer a liquid product, and while the taste isn't so great, adding your bitters to a small spray bottle and spraying it into your mouth before meals can help with the taste.

ABOUT THE AUTHOR

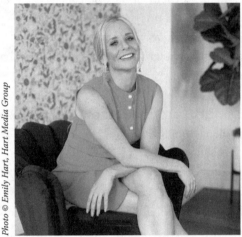

Photo © Emily Hart, Hart Media Group

Megan Hansen, a registered dietitian nutritionist, is the founder and CEO of Metabolism Makeover—a virtual nutrition-coaching business with a focus on weight loss and metabolic health. With a community of almost 40 dietitians and over 6,000 past and present clients, Hansen's company is dedicated to helping clients learn how to change their relationship with food so that they can lose the weight, *and* the food anxiety, and keep it off for good. As a speaker and industry leader, Megan has been featured in *Eating Well, Martha Stewart Living* magazine, and *The Skinny Confidential*. She lives in Atlanta, Georgia. Visit her website at www.metabolismmakeover.co.